Nursing care

In

Cardiac Surgery

The Complete Guide

ALEXANDRE CAREWELL

2

Table of contents

« *In the hands of a heart surgeon, a heart is not just an organ, but the symbol of a second chance with every beat.* »

Chapter 1:
INTRODUCTION
CARDIAC SURGERY

History and development of cardiac surgery

The history of cardiac surgery is both fascinating and a testament to mankind's incredible ability to push back the boundaries of science and medicine to save lives. Delving into the past, we discover that the first interventions on the heart were considered an impassable frontier, an area of the human body that was called "the forbidden zone". The complexity and sensitivity of the heart long stood in the way of direct surgery.

In the early 20th century, brave pioneers dared to approach this mysterious organ, performing simple operations, often in last-chance circumstances. However, the real breakthrough came with the development of the heart-lung machine in the 1950s. This revolutionary device enabled blood flow to be diverted temporarily, giving surgeons a window of opportunity to operate on the stationary heart.

This innovation opened the doors to modern cardiac surgery, leading to a series of rapid advances. Aorto-coronary bypass, valve surgery and even heart transplantation became feasible. Lives that would once have been lost to heart defects or advanced heart disease have been saved.

Over the decades, cardiac surgery has continued to evolve, incorporating new technologies and techniques. Minimally invasive surgery, for example, has made it possible to perform major procedures through small incisions, significantly reducing recovery times and complications. Advanced imaging methods, innovative materials for prostheses and implants, and improved protocols for pre- and post-operative care have also played a key role.

Today, cardiac surgery, once seen as a miracle, has become a standard procedure in many hospitals around the world. Cardiac surgeons, armed with in-depth knowledge and cutting-edge technology, continue to expand the horizons of what is possible, while always remembering the bold pioneers who came before them. And while the challenges persist, the future of cardiac surgery looks bright, offering the hope of new innovations and even more remarkable cures.

The challenges and the complexity Of cardiac surgery

Cardiac surgery, the cornerstone of modern medicine, is fraught with considerable challenges and complexity inherent in the organ it treats: the heart. This vital organ, the driving force behind life, represents a constant challenge for surgeons because of its importance and its delicate mechanics.

One of the first issues is undoubtedly the risk associated with any operation on such a vital organ. A simple error, a slight misalignment or a minor complication can have fatal consequences. This reality places a huge responsibility on the surgeon's shoulders, where every decision counts and the margin for error is minimal.

The technical complexity of the procedures is another major aspect. Surgeons must have an in-depth knowledge of cardiac anatomy, understand the subtleties of the different tissues, veins, arteries and valves, and master the use of cutting-edge equipment. The arrival of new technologies, such as robot-assisted surgery and advanced imaging techniques, while bringing considerable advantages, also requires specific training and skills.

The rapid evolution of medical knowledge and technology also means that surgeons need to be constantly up to date. Yesterday's protocols may be obsolete tomorrow, replaced by new, more effective or safer approaches.

What's more, cardiac surgery does not stop at the operation itself. Equally important are the pre-operative care, which is crucial for preparing the patient and minimising risks, and the post-operative phase, which is essential for ensuring optimum recovery and preventing complications. Collaboration with other health professionals - cardiologists, anaesthetists, specialist nurses, physiotherapists - is therefore essential.

Finally, there is the ethical and human issue. Beyond their technical skills, cardiac surgeons are often faced with difficult decisions: when to operate, when to choose a less invasive alternative, when, unfortunately, to recognise that surgery can no longer help. At such times, the ability to communicate compassionately, weigh up the pros and cons, and respect the patient's wishes and dignity is fundamental.

Cardiac surgery, while a field of medical excellence, remains a delicate art, where science, technique, ethics and humanity must constantly intertwine to offer patients the very best.

The importance of the nurse
in this speciality

Cardiac surgery, with its complexities and challenges, requires a dedicated and skilled medical team in which each member plays a crucial role. In this context, the nurse, often perceived as the surgeon's discreet but essential shadow, takes on particular importance.

From the outset, the cardiac surgery nurse is one of the first points of contact for the patient. They gather essential medical information, assess the patient's condition and help to put the care plan in place. This first impression, this ability to reassure and establish a relationship of trust, can have a significant impact on the patient's overall experience.

The nurse also plays a pivotal role during the operation itself, although this is often outside the operating theatre. They prepare the patient, ensure that all the necessary medical devices are ready and make sure that safety protocols are followed to the letter.

After surgery, it is often the nurse who takes care of the patient during the crucial first moments in the recovery room. They monitor vital signs, manage pain, detect any complications and are ready to intervene in an emergency. In the days that follow, the nurse continues to monitor the patient's progress, administering medication, changing dressings, guiding the patient through physiotherapy and ensuring a smooth transition to recovery at home.

In addition to these clinical responsibilities, the cardiac surgery nurse plays an essential role in patient and family education. They inform them about the nature of the operation, post-operative care, signs of complications and the stages of recovery. This education is vital if the patient is to understand, actively participate in their recovery and adopt behaviours that will benefit their long-term heart health.

But beyond technical and educational skills, it is perhaps in the human aspect that nurses shine brightest. For many, cardiac surgery is a frightening, emotionally-charged experience. The nurse offers comfort, a listening ear and psychological support, often becoming the reassuring hand to shake or the shoulder to lean on.

So, in the precise, coordinated ballet of cardiac surgery, the nurse is much more than a simple auxiliary: he or she is a cornerstone, ensuring the patient's well-being at every stage, guaranteeing that, beyond science and technique, the human element always remains at the heart of the therapeutic approach.

Chapter 2:
ANATOMY AND
CARDIAC PHYSIOLOGY

Understanding the heart : structure and functions

At the heart of our circulatory system lies an exceptional organ, the heart, whose precise and constant mechanics ensure the distribution of blood throughout our body. To understand the complexity of cardiac surgery, it is essential to begin with a detailed exploration of this fascinating organ.

Core structure :
The heart is a hollow muscle divided into four chambers: two atria (left and right) and two ventricles (left and right). These chambers are separated by partitions: the atrial septum between the atria and the ventricular septum between the ventricles.

Blood flow through these chambers is regulated by four heart valves:

- The mitral valve: between the left atrium and the left ventricle.
- The tricuspid valve: between the right atrium and the right ventricle.
- The pulmonary valve: at the exit of the right ventricle towards the pulmonary artery.
- The aortic valve: at the exit of the left ventricle towards the aorta.

Functions of the heart :

- **Pumping**: The heart acts like a pump, circulating blood throughout the body. The left ventricle pumps oxygenated blood throughout the body via the aorta, while the right ventricle sends deoxygenated blood to the lungs via the pulmonary artery.

Oxygenation: The right atrium receives deoxygenated blood from the veins and directs it to the right ventricle. From there, it is sent to the lungs for oxygenation. Once oxygenated, the blood returns to the heart, entering the left atrium before being pumped to the left ventricle and then to the rest of the body.

Rhythmicity: The heart has an intrinsic electrical system that ensures regular contraction. The sino-atrial node (SAN), located in the right atrium, is the heart's natural pacemaker. It generates electrical impulses that travel through the atria, then to the atrioventricular node (AVN) and finally to the ventricles, triggering muscle contraction.

The heart and circulatory system :
The heart works closely with the blood vessels to form the circulatory system. This system is divided into two main circuits:

Pulmonary circuit: where blood is sent to the lungs for oxygenation.

Systemic circuit: where oxygenated blood is transported to all the other organs and tissues of the body.

The heart is a marvel of biological engineering, a robust yet delicate machine that sustains life within us with every beat. Its complex structure and vital functions require a deep understanding for those seeking to intervene surgically. And even for ordinary mortals, an appreciation of this amazing organ can lead to healthier lifestyle choices and better heart health.

Common cardiac pathologies

Heart diseases are many and varied, affecting millions of people worldwide. These diseases can affect the very structure of the heart, its pumping capacity, or the electrical system that controls its rhythm. Here is a list of common heart conditions:

Coronary heart disease (or atherosclerosis) :
> This is the most common cause of heart disease. It is due to the accumulation of atheromatous plaques (lipid deposits) on the walls of the coronary arteries, reducing the supply of oxygen to the heart muscle.
> Can lead to angina pectoris or myocardial infarction (heart attack).

Heart failure :
> Occurs when the heart does not pump blood as efficiently as it should.
> May result from other heart conditions such as myocardial infarction or high blood pressure.

Cardiomyopathies :
> These are diseases of the heart muscle itself.
> These can be due to genetic causes, infections, toxins or metabolic diseases.

Valvulopathies :
> Conditions affecting the heart valves, which may be narrowed (stenosis) or fail to close properly (insufficiency or regurgitation).

Heart rhythm disorders (arrhythmias) :
> Abnormal heart rate or rhythm.
> Examples: atrial fibrillation, ventricular tachycardia, ventricular fibrillation, heart block.

- Congenital heart defects :
    - Structural abnormalities of the heart present from birth, such as tetralogy of Fallot or ventricular septal defect.
- Pericarditis :
    - Inflammation of the thin membrane surrounding the heart, the pericardium.
    - Can be caused by infection, trauma or other medical conditions.
- Endocarditis :
    - Inflammation of the inner lining of the heart, often caused by a bacterial infection.
- Hypertensive heart disease :
    - Heart problems caused by high blood pressure, which can affect the heart, the arteries, or both.
- Ischaemic heart disease :
    - Caused by a reduction in the blood supply to the heart muscle, generally due to coronary atherosclerosis.

These conditions, although common, vary considerably in their symptoms, causes and treatments. Numerous medical, surgical and lifestyle interventions can help to manage, treat or prevent these conditions. Understanding and knowledge of these conditions is essential for anyone working in cardiology or cardiac surgery.

Cardiology diagnostic techniques and equipment

Cardiology, as a medical speciality, relies on a wide range of diagnostic techniques and equipment to assess heart function, identify heart disease and determine the best therapeutic approach. Here is an overview of the techniques and equipment commonly used in the field:

Electrocardiogram (ECG) :
> Measures the electrical activity of the heart.

> Used to detect arrhythmias, myocardial infarction and other abnormalities.

Echocardiography (echo) :
> Uses ultrasound waves to produce images of the heart in motion.

> It can assess the size, shape and function of the ventricles and valves, and detect heart malformations.

Stress test :
> The patient performs physical activity (often on a treadmill) while his or her cardiac activity is monitored.

> Used to detect coronary artery disease.

Holter ECG :
> A portable device that records the electrical activity of the heart over a prolonged period (often 24 hours).

> Used to detect intermittent arrhythmias.

Cardiac magnetic resonance imaging test (cardiac MRI) :
> Uses magnetic fields to produce detailed images of the heart.

> Can detect cardiomyopathy, heart tumours and other abnormalities.

Cardiac computed tomography (cardiac CT) :
> A form of X-ray that provides detailed cross-sectional images of the heart.

> Often used to visualise coronary arteries and detect calcium deposits.

Cardiac catheterisation (or coronary angiography) :
> A catheter is inserted into an artery and guided to the heart.

> Allows pressures to be measured, blood flow to be analysed and a dye to be injected to visualise the coronary arteries.

- Coronary angiography :
  - A specific   form of cardiac catheterisation in which a dye is injected to visualise the coronary arteries using X-rays.
- Nuclear stress test :
  - A small quantity   of radioactive substance is injected, and the patient then undergoes a stress test.
  - Images are captured to assess blood flow to the heart during exercise.
- Tilt-test :
  - The patient is placed on a table which changes angle.
  - Used to diagnose the causes of unexplained fainting.
- Electrophysiology (EP) :
  - Study of the heart's electrical circuits.
  - Allows the source of arrhythmias to be located and the best treatment to be determined.
- Cardiac event monitor :
  - A portable device that can be activated by the patient when they experience symptoms.
  - Records electrical activity during these episodes.

These diagnostic tools, often used in combination, provide cardiologists with a detailed overview of cardiac function and possible diseases. They are essential for guiding therapeutic decisions and improving outcomes for patients suffering from cardiac pathologies.

Chapter 3:
BEFORE THE OPERATION -
THE PRE-OPERATIVE ROLE
THE NURSE

Pre-operative patient assessment

The pre-operative assessment of a patient undergoing cardiac surgery is a crucial stage in ensuring the success of the operation and minimising the risks. This comprehensive assessment encompasses clinical, functional, psychological and social aspects. Its aim is to identify potential problems that could influence the course of the surgery and post-operative recovery.

- Clinical evaluation :
  - **Medical history:** medical history, previous surgery, current medication and allergies.
  - **Physical examination**: Assessment of general condition, cardiac function (auscultation, palpation), pulmonary function and other body systems.
- Diagnostic tests :
  - **Electrocardiogram (ECG):** Analysis of the electrical activity of the heart.
  - **Echocardiography**: Assessment of cardiac function and structure.
  - **Chest X-ray**: Examination of the lungs and the size/shape of the heart.
  - **Blood tests**: Assessment of renal function, liver function, electrolyte levels, complete blood count and coagulation.
  - **Exercise stress test**: Evaluation of cardiac capacity during exercise.

Cardiac catheterisation: If necessary, to assess the condition of the coronary arteries and heart chambers.

Functional assessment :

Assessment of the patient's ability to carry out daily activities.

Identification of functional limitations that may require post-operative rehabilitation.

Psychosocial assessment :

Assessment of the patient's psychological state and ability to understand and adhere to post-operative recommendations.

Consideration of family or social support available after surgery.

Nutritional assessment :

Assessment of nutritional status to detect any deficiencies.

Advice and recommendations for optimising pre-operative nutrition.

Assessment of anaesthetic risks :

Consultation with the anaesthetist to assess the specific risks associated with anaesthesia.

Discussion of possible anaesthetic methods and management of post-operative pain.

Evaluation of other systems :

Pulmonary function, kidney tests, neurological assessment, if necessary, depending on the patient's history and the anticipated risks of surgery.

Discussion with the patient and family:

Presentation of the risks, benefits and alternatives to surgery.

Obtaining informed consent.

This exhaustive pre-operative assessment aims to give the patient the best chance of surgical success while reducing potential complications. It requires close collaboration between cardiologists, surgeons, anaesthetists, nurses and other healthcare professionals to ensure optimal patient care.

Patient education : mental and physical preparation

Patient education prior to cardiac surgery is a fundamental pillar of the pre-operative process. Surgery, especially on an organ as vital as the heart, can be an overwhelming experience for many patients. The emotional, psychological and physical issues involved demand careful preparation.

On the one hand, mental preparation is essential. It enables the patient to understand the nature of the operation, its benefits, risks and long-term implications. By acquiring this knowledge, patients can gradually overcome their fear, anxiety and any other feelings of uncertainty. Medical teams, through information sessions, educational brochures or testimonials from other patients who have had a similar experience, can greatly help to demystify surgery. It is also crucial to encourage patients to ask questions, express their concerns and discuss their feelings with their loved ones or healthcare professionals.

Physical preparation is just as essential. It covers several aspects. Firstly, it involves optimising the patient's physical condition to encourage rapid post-operative recovery. This may involve endurance, muscle strengthening or breathing exercises, always adapted to the patient's individual situation. Secondly, it is vital to make patients aware of the importance of a balanced diet to boost the immune system and reduce the risk of post-operative infections. In addition, education sessions can be organised to teach the patient pain management techniques, how to move around after the operation and how to identify and report any complications.

Patient education is a continuous, two-way process. It involves close collaboration between the patient, his or her family and the medical team. By arming patients with knowledge, equipping them with the necessary tools and encouraging them to play an active role in their care, we can give them the best possible chance of success, both mentally and physically.

Coordination with the surgical team

Coordination with the surgical team is one of the most crucial stages in the management of a cardiac surgery patient. It guarantees not only the success of the operation, but also the safety and well-being of the patient. This coordination is akin to a medical ballet, with each professional playing a key role, orchestrated with precision to ensure total harmony during the operation and in the post-operative period.

Firstly, there is the cardiac surgeon, the master of the operation, who establishes the surgical plan based on the patient's diagnosis. His coordination with the team is essential to ensure that every stage of the surgery goes according to plan. He or she must also work closely with the anaesthetist, who plays a crucial role in ensuring that the patient remains stable during the operation. The anaesthetist must be informed of every stage of the operation so that he can adapt his anaesthetic strategy accordingly.

Then there are the operating theatre nurses. They prepare the operating field, assist the surgeon by providing the necessary instruments and ensure that the environment remains sterile. Their role is essential to the smooth running of the operation and to minimising the risk of infection.

Outside the operating theatre, the coordination team also plays a crucial role. This includes the clinical nurses, who prepare the patient for surgery, educate them about the procedure and look after them after the operation, as well as the medical assistants, who manage appointments, tests and the logistics associated with the patient's stay in hospital.

It is also essential to coordinate with specialists such as cardiologists, radiologists and other health professionals who can provide valuable information about the patient's condition and the best treatment protocols to follow.

Finally, communication with the patient and his family is an equally vital aspect of this coordination. The surgical team must ensure that the patient understands the nature of the operation, the associated risks, and the stages involved in post-operative recovery.

Overall, coordination with the surgical team is a complex process that requires open communication, mutual respect between professionals and a constant focus on the patient's well-being. Each member of the team brings their own expertise to the table, and it is by working together, in a synchronised way, that they can guarantee the best outcome for the patient.

Chapter 4:
IN THE OPERATING THEATRE - ALONGSIDE THE SURGEON

Sterile preparation and setting up instruments

Sterile preparation and placement of instruments are critical steps in cardiac surgery. They ensure patient safety, by preventing the risk of infection, and make the operation run more smoothly for the surgical team. Although these steps may seem routine to seasoned professionals, they require extreme concentration and rigorous methodology.

Sterile preparation begins long before the patient enters the operating theatre. It requires meticulous disinfection of the room, the equipment and, of course, the patient himself. Every surface, every tool, every pair of hands that comes into contact with the operating field must be sterilised. This involves rigorous cleaning of the room, antiseptic washing of staff hands and forearms, the use of sterile surgical gowns and the use of surgical drapes to isolate the operating area.

Positioning the instruments is also an art in itself. Each instrument has a specific function, and its immediate availability can make the difference between a smooth operation and a more complicated situation. Instruments are generally placed on sterile trays, in an arrangement that respects their order of use or function. The operating theatre nurse, or surgical assistant, knows these instruments inside out, and knows exactly where each tool is, so they can provide it to the surgeon in a fraction of a second when requested.

The process of sterile preparation and instrument placement is governed by strict protocols, which define each stage. These protocols are the result of decades of surgical experience and have been developed to maximise patient safety while providing the surgical team with an optimal working environment.

Sterility must be maintained throughout the operation. This means that every movement, every gesture, must be carried out with the utmost care. If an instrument is dropped or the sterile field is compromised in any way, immediate action must be taken to correct the situation and protect the patient.

Sterile preparation and instrument placement are silent but absolutely crucial steps in surgery. They demonstrate the surgical team's dedication to ensuring the patient's safety and well-being, while working with the utmost efficiency and precision.

Continuous patient monitoring

Continuous patient monitoring during and after cardiac surgery is a vital part of medical care. It aims not only to ensure the patient's safety, but also to detect early any complications or changes in their condition that may require intervention. In the dynamic and often unpredictable environment of cardiac surgery, rigorous monitoring is key to ensuring that patients receive the best possible care at every stage of their recovery.

During surgery, the anaesthetist plays a central role by constantly monitoring the patient's vital signs. These include heart rate, blood pressure, oxygen saturation and other specific parameters such as the level of anaesthetic. Any fluctuation in these parameters may indicate a problem that requires immediate intervention. The anaesthetist uses a range of equipment, including heart monitors and pulse oximeters, to monitor the patient's condition in real time.

After surgery, when the patient is transferred to intensive care or a cardiac surgery unit, continuous monitoring remains essential. Cardiac monitors constantly track the heart's electrical activity, while other devices measure blood pressure, respiratory rate and body temperature. Nurses, on the front line of this monitoring, observe and interpret the data, while regularly assessing the patient for any signs of distress or complications.

But monitoring doesn't stop at machines and screens. It also includes repeated clinical assessments to ensure that the patient is waking up correctly from anaesthesia, that neurological function is intact, that surgical wounds are healing as expected and that there are no signs of infection. Pain, discomfort, confusion or other symptoms reported by the patient themselves are also valuable indicators that can guide the medical team to possible problems.

Communication between the medical team is vital in this monitoring process. Nurses, doctors, physiotherapists and other specialists constantly exchange information about the patient's condition, ensuring that each professional is kept up to date with the latest developments.

Continuous patient monitoring in cardiac surgery is a complex ballet, where cutting-edge technology and clinical skills combine to provide an invaluable safety net. It is thanks to this constant attention and unfailing vigilance that complications can be detected early and managed proactively, maximising each patient's chances of recovery and success.

Surgical assistance : the key moments

Surgical assistance in cardiac surgery is a precise and synchronised dance, where every action, every decision, every gesture counts. This coordination between the lead surgeon and his assistant is crucial to the success of the operation and the well-being of the patient. Here's a look at the key moments in surgical assistance in cardiac surgery.

1. Preparation before the operation :
Even before the patient is brought into the operating theatre, the surgical assistant works closely with the surgeon to prepare for the operation. This involves reviewing the patient's medical file, discussing the techniques to be used, and preparing the necessary instruments and equipment.

2. Positioning the patient :
Once the patient is asleep, the assistant helps to position him or her correctly on the operating table. This step is crucial to ensure optimum access to the operating area while protecting the patient from possible injury or complications.

3. Surgical opening :
During the initial incision and access to the heart, the assistant plays a crucial role by holding back the tissue, using retractors to give the surgeon a clear field of vision, and anticipating the surgeon's needs to facilitate access.

4. Critical moments in the intervention :
During delicate phases, such as bypass surgery or valve repair, the assistant is there to provide the necessary instruments, aspirate fluids or suture. Every gesture is coordinated, every action anticipated.

5. Closing :
After the main cardiac procedure has been completed, the assistant helps to close the surgical area. This often involves placing sutures, checking haemostasis (to ensure there is no bleeding) and applying dressings.

6. Final instrument count :
To ensure the patient's safety, the surgical assistant, together with the ward nurse, makes sure that all the instruments used during the operation are accounted for and that no objects have been left inside the patient.

7. Transfer and communication :
After the operation, the surgical assistant plays a key role in transferring the patient to the recovery room or intensive care unit. They are also essential for communicating the details of the operation to the post-operative care team.

These key moments highlight the indispensable role of the surgical assistant in cardiac surgery. His or her ability to anticipate the surgeon's needs, react quickly to unforeseen circumstances and work in harmony with the entire operating team is essential to guarantee the best possible outcome for the patient.

Chapter 5:
AFTER THE OPERATION -
POST-OPERATIVE CARE

Immediate post-operative monitoring:
vital signs
and potential complications

Immediate post-operative monitoring after cardiac surgery is a critical phase where maximum attention must be paid to the patient. The first few hours after such an operation are essential for the rapid detection and treatment of any complications. The patient's vital signs and physiological parameters are meticulously monitored, reflecting the functioning of the body and the newly operated heart.

1. Vital signs :
   - **Heart rate:** Constant monitoring is carried out to detect any arrhythmia or irregularity in the heart rhythm.
   - **Blood pressure:** Blood pressure must be stable. High or low blood pressure could indicate bleeding or weakness of the heart muscle respectively.
   - **Oxygen saturation:** A drop could indicate a problem with lung or heart function.
   - **Respiratory rate:** This is monitored, especially if the patient is still intubated or is showing signs of respiratory distress.
   - **Body temperature:** Fever could indicate an infection, while hypothermia could be the result of the extracorporeal circulation used during surgery.
2. Potential complications to watch out for :
   - **Cardiac tamponade:** An accumulation of fluid in the pericardium that can compress the heart.

- **Haemorrhage:** Blood loss is common after cardiac surgery. Monitoring of drains and drainage devices is essential.
- **Thromboembolism:** Clots can form and cause a stroke or pulmonary embolism.
- **Renal insufficiency:** The kidneys may be affected by surgery or extracorporeal circulation. Urea and creatinine levels are monitored.
- **Graft malfunction:** After a heart transplant, the function of the new heart must be monitored.

3. Other parameters to be monitored :
- **Pain:** Managing patients' pain is crucial to their recovery.
- **Lung function:** Auscultation and measurement of lung capacity help to detect any respiratory complications.
- **Neurological signs:** Consciousness, ability to move, speech and other neurological signs are assessed to detect possible brain damage.

4. Communication with the patient :

It is essential to reassure patients, inform them about the operation and answer any questions they may have. This communication strengthens the patient's trust in the medical team and facilitates their cooperation during the monitoring phase.

Immediate post-operative monitoring is a key stage in the management of patients who have undergone cardiac surgery. The speed with which potential complications are detected and managed during this period can greatly influence the patient's outcome and recovery.

Pain management and patient comfort

Pain management and patient comfort after cardiac surgery are central to optimal recovery. Poorly controlled pain can hamper healing, increase the risk of post-operative complications and adversely affect the patient's quality of life. Here is an overview of this management, combining medical techniques, nursing care and complementary approaches.

1. Pain assessment :
Above all, it is crucial to assess the patient's pain on a regular basis. Pain scales, such as the visual analogue scale (VAS) or the numerical scale, can be used. The patient's expression, posture and behaviour are also key indicators.

2. Analgesic drugs :

- **Non-opioid analgesics:** Such as paracetamol or non-steroidal anti-inflammatory drugs (NSAIDs), used for mild to moderate pain.
- **Opioids:** such as morphine or fentanyl, prescribed for moderate to severe pain. They require careful monitoring because of their side effects.
- **Adjuvant medications:** Such as anticonvulsants or antidepressants, which can be used to treat certain neuropathic pains.

3. Non-pharmacological techniques :

- **Thermotherapy:** Applying heat or cold can relieve pain.
- **Massage:** Can help relax muscles and improve circulation.
- **Relaxation and deep breathing:** help reduce tension and anxiety.
- **Early mobilisation:** Encouraging the patient to move and walk can help prevent stiffness and improve circulation.

4. Patient comfort :

   Positioning: Ensure a comfortable position in bed and regularly change the patient's position to prevent pressure sores.

   Hygiene: Regular care of the skin and mucous membranes, as well as mouthwash, can improve comfort.

   Nutrition: The right diet can help with convalescence and boost well-being.

5. Patient education :

   • It is essential to inform patients about the importance of reporting their pain, and about the drugs prescribed and their potential side-effects. Patients must also be informed of the non-medicinal techniques available to them.

6. Regular monitoring :

   • The patient's pain and comfort must be reassessed regularly to ensure that interventions are effective and to adjust the care plan if necessary.

7. Complementary approaches :

   • Techniques such as acupuncture, movement therapy and music can also be explored, depending on the patient's needs and preferences.

The management of pain and comfort after cardiac surgery is multi-dimensional and requires close collaboration between the patient, the healthcare team and relatives. Effective management can speed up recovery, improve patient satisfaction and reduce the risk of complications.

Patient education for home recovery

Patient education for recovery at home after cardiac surgery is crucial to ensure a safe and effective recovery. The first few weeks at home require special attention for both the patient and their carers. Going home is a moment to look forward to, but it can also be a source of anxiety. Preparing the patient is therefore essential.

1. Physical activities :

    Progressive mobilisation: Patients should gradually increase their level of activity, starting with short daily walks.

    Limitations: Avoid heavy lifting and strenuous activities for the first few weeks.

    Rehabilitation: If necessary, a cardiac rehabilitation programme may be recommended to strengthen the heart and improve endurance.

2. Wound care :

    Monitoring: Examine the wound daily for signs of infection such as redness, oozing or sutures pulling apart.

    Cleaning: Follow the instructions given for cleaning the wound and changing dressings.

3. Medicines :

    Compliance with prescriptions: Take all medicines as prescribed, without interruption, unless otherwise advised by your doctor.

    Side-effects: Be aware of any side-effects and know when to seek medical advice.

4. Nutrition :

    Balanced diet: Adopt a heart-healthy diet, rich in fruit, vegetables and whole grains and low in salt and saturated fats.

    Limiting fluids: Depending on your doctor's advice, you may need to limit your water intake.

5. Warning signs :

    • Inform the patient of any symptoms requiring urgent medical attention, such as chest pain, abnormal breathlessness, palpitations or oedema.

6. Medical follow-up :

    Consultations: Keep all post-operative appointments with the surgeon and cardiologist.

Check-up: Regular check-ups, such as blood tests or electrocardiograms, may be scheduled.

7. Emotional well-being :

Support: Encourage patients to express their feelings and concerns. Cardiac surgery can have an emotional impact.

Support groups: Some patients benefit from sharing their experiences with others who have undergone a similar operation.

8. Other advice :

Smoking: It's essential to stop smoking to protect your heart.

Sleep: Make sure you get enough rest, avoiding prolonged naps which can disrupt night-time sleep.

9. Implications for carers :

Relatives need to be trained to provide the necessary care and to monitor symptoms. They play a key role in providing emotional and practical support.

Recovery at home after cardiac surgery is an important stage that requires preparation, education and support. With the right tools and information, patients can expect a safe return home and a gradual resumption of their activities.

Chapter 6:
PSYCHOLOGICAL CHALLENGES AND EMOTIONAL

Understanding stress and patient anxiety

The medical journey, particularly when it involves operations as significant as cardiac surgery, is punctuated by moments of uncertainty and anxiety for the patient. Stress and anxiety, although universal to some extent, can vary in intensity and nature from one individual to another. Understanding these feelings is essential to providing holistic care.

1. Origins of stress and anxiety :
- **Fear of the unknown:** Not knowing what to expect before, during and after surgery can be a source of anxiety.
- **Fear of pain:** Post-operation pain or even pain associated with preliminary examinations is a common concern.
- **Concerns about results:** Fear that surgery will not have the desired effects or will lead to complications.
- **Financial implications:** The cost of treatment, medication and post-operative care can be stressful.

2. Physiological signs :
Stress and anxiety can manifest as symptoms such as :
- Heart palpitations.
- An increase in blood pressure.
- Sleep disorders.
- Stomach ache or digestive problems.

3. Consequences for recovery :
High levels of anxiety can :
- Extend healing time.

Affect the patient's ability to follow medical recommendations.

Exacerbate the pain felt.

4. Listening and communication strategies :

Ask questions: Asking patients regularly how they are feeling helps to identify their concerns.

Reassurance: Providing clear and precise information can help demystify surgery and reduce anxiety.

Involve: Involving patients in decisions relating to their care means that they play an active role in their care.

5. Stress management techniques :

Relaxation techniques: Deep breathing, meditation or visualisation can help manage anxiety.

Cognitive-behavioural therapy: This approach can help to identify and modify negative thoughts.

Psychological support: A consultation with a psychologist or psychiatrist may be beneficial.

Support groups: Sharing your experience with other patients can provide a sense of solidarity.

6. Implications for relatives :

It is important to recognise that a patient's anxiety can also affect those close to them. Supporting them and educating them about how the patient is feeling is crucial to an integrated approach to care.

Recognising and addressing patient stress and anxiety is an essential aspect of pre- and post-operative care. Empathetic, holistic care not only humanises the medical journey but can also improve clinical outcomes and patient satisfaction.

Providing emotional support

Providing emotional support to a patient, particularly in a medical context, is just as vital as physiological care. The road to recovery is not simply paved with drugs and surgery, but is also deeply rooted in the psychological dimension of well-being. The weight of emotions, whether anxiety about a diagnosis, fear of a procedure or distress caused by pain, can often overshadow the physical ailments themselves.

The role of the medical staff, and more broadly the people around the patient, is essential in this support process. Offering an attentive ear, being present and reassuring, can make all the difference. In this delicate ballet of emotions, the simple act of holding a patient's hand or offering words of encouragement can lighten the burden of their worries. But this support is not just about gestures or words; it's also about creating an environment conducive to serenity and trust.

Psychological consultations, relaxation and meditation sessions, and staff training in empathic communication are all valuable tools. Support groups, where patients share their experiences, can also provide a safe space where emotions are not only acknowledged but also valued.

But emotional support does not stop at the hospital or clinic. Family and friends have a major role to play. Their presence, understanding and patience can help patients feel grounded, supported and loved, creating a safety net around them.

The emotional dimension of medical care is not simply an adjunct; it is intrinsically linked to the way in which patients heal, perceive their illness and find their way back to a full and rewarding life. Recognising, valuing and responding to emotional needs is therefore a fundamental step in any comprehensive medical care.

Taking care of your own mental health

Taking care of our own mental health is not just a luxury, it's a vital necessity. In a world where the pace of life, daily challenges and societal demands seem endless, paying particular attention to our psychological well-being is essential for a balanced and fulfilled life.

Recognising our own emotions is the first step towards taking charge of our mental health. Each of us, at one time or another, may feel stress, anxiety, sadness or other emotions. These feelings are not a sign of weakness; they are a reflection of our experiences, our challenges and our humanity. Accepting them, without judgement, helps us to better understand what we are going through and to find appropriate solutions.

Lifestyle habits also play a crucial role. A balanced diet, regular exercise and quality sleep all have a positive influence on our state of mind. The link between body and mind is inextricable, and taking care of one invariably benefits the other.

Moments of relaxation and rejuvenation are essential. Whether through meditation, reading, the arts or simply a walk in nature, it's essential to take time to disconnect, refocus and recharge our emotional batteries.

Dialogue and sharing can provide a lifeline in difficult times. Discussing our concerns with friends, family or professionals can help to put things into perspective, find support and untangle certain emotions.

Education and awareness are also key. Understanding the warning signs of mental disorders, knowing what resources are available and keeping abreast of the latest advances in mental health can help prevent and effectively manage psychological challenges.

Let's not forget that **asking for help** is not a sign of weakness, but of strength. In some cases, consulting a mental health professional, whether a therapist, counsellor or psychiatrist, may be the best way to tackle and overcome obstacles.

Taking care of our own mental health is an ongoing journey of understanding, acceptance and proactivity. It's a commitment to ourselves that allows us not only to navigate through life's storms, but also to fully savour its moments of serenity.

Chapter 7:
WORKING AS PART OF A TEAM
IN CARDIAC SURGERY

Communicating effectively with surgeons, anaesthetists and other team members

Communication is the vital artery that irrigates the entire medical process, and it takes on a particularly crucial dimension within a surgical team. The complexity and precision required in cardiac surgery make communication a non-negotiable element in patient safety and well-being.

Navigating the dynamic and demanding landscape of the operating theatre requires a remarkable mastery of language, gestures and listening skills. Understanding the nuances of each specialist, whether surgeon or anaesthetist, is essential to anticipating their needs and acting accordingly. The exchange of information must be clear, concise and, above all, timely. It's not just a question of relaying messages, but of understanding the subtleties behind each request or indication.

Mutual trust between each member of the team is the cement of this communication. Each professional, aware of his or her role and responsibility, must also recognise and value the expertise of others. It is in this trust that the ability to ask questions, seek clarification or even make suggestions lies.

Synergy with anaesthetists, for example, is vital. Their interventions, which go far beyond simple sedation, require close collaboration to guarantee patient comfort and safety. Constant, fluid dialogue ensures that vital parameters are maintained, pain is managed and any complications are immediately identified and treated.

Moreover, communication is not limited to the critical moments of the operation. Pre-operative meetings, where the details and strategies of the operation are discussed, are just as crucial. These are the times when an action plan is drawn up, potential obstacles are identified and the team is aligned on common objectives.

In addition to words, it is also important to be attentive to what is not said, to gestures, tone of voice and the general atmosphere of the operating theatre. In an environment where every second counts, a simple facial expression or gesture can convey a vital message.

Communicating effectively with surgeons, anaesthetists and other team members is a delicate dance of respect, listening and understanding. It is this harmony, this symphony of interactions, that ensures that every patient receives the highest quality of care.

The role of the nurse
in multidisciplinary meetings

The role of the nurse in multidisciplinary meetings is much more than that of a simple participant. They are the bridge between the patient and the medical team, bringing a unique perspective that encompasses both the clinical and emotional needs of the patient. In these meetings, where various specialists come together to discuss care, the nurse plays several essential roles.

Firstly, nurses are often the first to witness patients' reactions to their treatment, whether physiological, emotional or psychosocial. They can provide invaluable information about the effectiveness of a treatment, any side effects, and the patient's concerns and feelings. This perspective is fundamental, as it ensures that the decisions taken are patient-centred and take account of the whole of the patient's experience.

What's more, thanks to their training and experience in the field, nurses can actively contribute to the clinical discussion. They can ask questions, propose solutions and even, in some cases, suggest alternatives based on their own expertise or on patient feedback. This contribution is all the more valuable if the nurse has in-depth knowledge of the patient's day-to-day reality.

Nurses also play a coordinating role. Being at the crossroads of many interactions - with the patient, family, doctors, therapists and other members of the care team - they are often best placed to ensure smooth communication between all stakeholders. They can clarify instructions, remind people of crucial information, or simply ensure that everyone is on the same wavelength.

Nurses also contribute their expertise in education and awareness-raising. Whether explaining a pathology, discussing the implications of a treatment or guiding a patient through pre-operative preparation, their ability to translate complex medical concepts into understandable terms is essential. In a multidisciplinary meeting, this skill can help to formulate care plans that not only meet clinical needs, but are also pragmatic and achievable.

The role of the nurse in these meetings goes beyond mere participation. They are a vital voice, a patient advocate, a key collaborator and an essential link in the care chain. In the vast orchestra of healthcare, the nurse is an invaluable musician, whose melody influences and enriches the overall symphony.

Managing emergency situations as a team

Managing emergency situations as a team is a carefully choreographed ballet, with each member playing a crucial role in a symphony of interdependent actions. In these moments of intensity, when every second counts, fluid coordination, clear communication and mutual trust are vital.

When an emergency situation arises, it is imperative that the medical team can instantly adopt an emergency dynamic. This means getting together quickly, assessing the situation accurately and making informed decisions in the patient's best interests.

The first step is assessment. Whether it's respiratory distress, cardiac arrest or sudden haemorrhage, it's essential to establish the seriousness of the situation quickly. It is often the nurse, because of his or her immediate proximity to the patient, who raises the alarm and begins the first interventions, while calling for help.

At such times, communication must be concise and precise. Every member of the team, whether doctor, nurse, anaesthetist or other healthcare professional, must be able to relay essential information in as few words as possible, while understanding and anticipating the needs of others. A look, a gesture or a simple word can be enough to convey a vital message.

Mutual trust is the secret ingredient that makes this complex machinery work. Each professional knows that his or her colleagues have been trained for these situations, and that they will act competently and diligently. It's not just a question of trust in technical skills, but also trust in each member's ability to remain calm, prioritise and collaborate under pressure.

Coordination is essential. In an emergency situation, there is no room for duplication of effort or hesitation. Every action must be orchestrated to avoid duplication and ensure optimum care. This may require a temporary hierarchy, with one person (often the most senior doctor or team leader) taking the reins and directing operations.

But beyond immediate action, managing emergency situations as a team also means knowing how to support each other. Emergencies are tough, both physically and emotionally. A word of encouragement, a gesture of support or even a simple glance can make a huge difference.

Faced with an emergency, the medical team becomes a united entity, with each member acting with unfailing determination and precision. It's a testament to the resilience, training and devotion of health professionals who, together, strive to save lives.

Chapter 8:
TECHNIQUES
AND SPECIFIC PROCEDURES
IN CARDIAC SURGERY

Open heart surgery
and minimally invasive surgery

Cardiac surgery, with its remarkable technological and medical advances, is a constantly evolving field. The spectrum ranges from open-heart surgery, a complex and invasive procedure, to minimally invasive surgery, which promises less trauma and faster recovery. Understanding these two poles of cardiac surgery is essential for nurses and all healthcare professionals involved in the care of cardiac patients.

Open Heart Surgery
a) Definition and process:
Open-heart surgery is a major operation in which the patient's chest is opened to allow direct access to the heart. It is generally performed under extracorporeal circulation, where a machine takes over the circulation of blood while the heart is stopped to allow surgery to take place.

b) Standard procedures:
Typical procedures include coronary bypass surgery, valve replacement and repair of congenital heart defects.

c) Role of the nurse:
Nurses play an essential role in patient preparation, intraoperative monitoring and intensive postoperative care. They must be highly qualified to manage potential

complications and ensure a stable and continuous recovery.

Minimally invasive surgery
a) Definition and process:
Minimally invasive surgery, also known as endoscopic cardiac surgery, is a more recent technique that seeks to minimise trauma by using much smaller incisions and often avoiding opening the chest completely.

b) Standard procedures:
It is frequently used for valvular procedures and certain interventions on the coronary arteries.

c) Role of the nurse:
In this context, nurses need to be familiar with the technology and specialised equipment, and able to offer appropriate post-operative care to promote rapid recovery and minimise complications.

Comparison and Considerations for the Future
a) Advantages and disadvantages:
Each type of surgery offers specific advantages and disadvantages. Open-heart surgery, although more invasive, allows direct and complete access, while minimally invasive surgery significantly reduces trauma and the length of hospitalisation.

b) Choice of Procedure:
The choice between these methods depends on a number of factors, including the specific nature of the cardiac pathology, the patient's general condition, and the technical capabilities of the surgical team.

c) Futurist evolution:
The future of cardiac surgery probably lies in the continued development of minimally invasive and robotic techniques,

while retaining open-heart surgery for the most complex cases.

In this dynamic and constantly evolving context, nurses, along with the entire medical team, must continually update their knowledge and skills, adapting and evolving with the science and technology of cardiac surgery to offer the best possible care to their patients.

Cardiac catheterisation and percutaneous interventions

Cardiac catheterisation and percutaneous interventions form a world of their own in the treatment of heart disease. These procedures, which are less invasive than open surgery, are often preferred for their less traumatic nature, faster recovery times and lower risk of complications.

Cardiac catheterisation
a) Definition and process:
Cardiac catheterisation is a diagnostic procedure that allows the functioning of the heart to be closely examined. A catheter is inserted into an artery (usually in the groin or arm) and guided to the heart. Once in place, the catheter can be used to measure the pressure in the various chambers of the heart or to inject a contrast product, enabling detailed imaging of the coronary arteries.

b) Applications:
This technique is often used to detect blockages or narrowing of the coronary arteries, to assess heart valves, or to diagnose other heart conditions.

c) Role of carers:
Preparing the patient by reassuring them about the nature of the procedure, monitoring the progress of the catheter, anticipating the needs of the cardiologist, and then

monitoring the insertion site for any sign of complication are crucial elements of the nurses' role.

Percutaneous procedures
a) Definition and process:
Percutaneous procedures, such as angioplasty, involve the use of catheters and other instruments to treat heart problems directly without the need for open surgery. In angioplasty, a balloon is inflated to open a blocked artery, and often a stent (a small metal tube) is deployed to keep the artery open.

b) Applications:
These procedures are commonly used to treat cardiac ischaemia, certain aneurysms and other vascular conditions. They can also be used to treat heart valve disease without the need for open surgery.

c) Role of carers:
The nurse must ensure adequate preparation of the patient, constant monitoring during the procedure, and specific post-procedural care. Pain management, monitoring of vital signs and observation of the insertion site for haemorrhage are essential.

Global Considerations
The advantages of percutaneous procedures include smaller incisions, shorter hospitalisation and generally faster recovery. However, they are not without risks, and a proper assessment is essential to determine the best approach for each patient.

As technology advances, these less invasive techniques continue to develop and improve, offering new treatment options for cardiac patients. For nurses and other healthcare professionals, keeping up to date with these advances and adapting to new techniques is essential to ensure optimal and safe care for their patients.

HEART TRANSPLANTATION: PROCESS AND POST-OPERATIVE CARE

Heart transplantation, an impressive medical achievement, is often the last treatment option for patients with end-stage heart failure. The process is complex and involves multidisciplinary care, before, during and after the operation. For nurses, a thorough understanding of the transplant process and post-operative requirements is crucial to ensure the patient's well-being and survival.

The heart transplant process
a) Evaluation and Selection:
Before a patient is considered for transplantation, an exhaustive assessment is carried out to ensure that they are both medically and psychologically fit. This assessment takes into account the severity of the heart failure, the prognosis without transplantation, and the patient's ability to adhere to the strict post-operative regimen.

b) Waiting for the donation:
Once a patient is approved for transplantation, they are placed on a waiting list for a suitable donor. During this period, the patient may require hospitalisation for cardiac support or other interventions to stabilise their condition.

c) The operation:
When a compatible heart is found, the patient is rapidly prepared for surgery. The transplant itself is a major operation in which the diseased heart is removed and replaced by the donor heart.

Post-operative care
a) Intensive surveillance:
After transplantation, the patient is usually placed in an intensive care unit where he or she is closely monitored for

possible complications, such as rejection of the new organ, infections or circulatory problems.

b) Discharge management:
One of the main concerns after a transplant is the risk of rejection of the new organ by the recipient's immune system. To prevent this, patients are given immunosuppressive drugs. Nurses play a key role in educating patients about the importance of these drugs and their possible side effects.

c) Rehabilitation:
The recovery process often involves rehabilitation to help the patient regain strength and endurance. Nurses help to coordinate and monitor this rehabilitation, ensuring that the patient makes progress without overloading the new heart.

d) Long-term monitoring:
Post-transplant monitoring is a lifelong commitment. Patients must see their doctors regularly and undergo tests to monitor the function of the new heart. Nurses, often the first point of contact for patients between these visits, must be vigilant for signs of complications or non-compliance with treatment.

e) Emotional support:
Heart transplantation is an emotionally charged experience. Nurses often play a supportive role, helping patients to manage anxiety, depression and the psychological challenges associated with such a procedure.

Heart transplantation, while offering a new chance at life, comes with its own set of challenges. Nurses, at the heart of transplant patient care, need to be equipped not only with medical knowledge but also with communication, empathy and support skills to help their patients through this life-changing period.

Chapter 9:
MANAGEMENT
SPECIFIC COMPLICATIONS

Post-operative arrhythmias

Post-operative arrhythmias are irregular heart rhythms that occur after heart surgery. They are common and can range from mild and temporary to severe and potentially fatal. Their origin is multifactorial, resulting from surgical trauma, electrolyte changes, ischaemia or inflammation. Understanding arrhythmias is essential for healthcare professionals, particularly nurses, to ensure optimal patient management.

Types of post-operative arrhythmia
a) Atrial fibrillation (AF):
It is the most common post-operative arrhythmia following heart surgery, particularly heart valve surgery. AF can increase the risk of stroke and often requires anticoagulant treatment.

b) Atrial flutter:
Similar to AF, atrial flutter involves rapid but more organised electrical activity in the atria. It can convert into AF or vice versa.

c) Heart blocks:
These can be atrioventricular blocks of varying degrees. In some cases, temporary or permanent implantation of a pacemaker may be necessary.

d) Ventricular tachycardia (VT):
Less common than AF but potentially more dangerous, VT can degenerate into ventricular fibrillation, a medical emergency.

56

Risk Factors

Factors that may contribute to post-operative arrhythmias include electrolyte imbalances (particularly potassium and magnesium), advanced age, pre-existing heart failure, hypertension, and the nature and duration of the surgery.

Taking charge

a) Surveillance:

Close monitoring is crucial. Patients are generally monitored continuously to detect any irregularities at an early stage.

b) Medication:

Anti-arrhythmic drugs, such as amiodarone, may be prescribed. Anticoagulants may also be necessary to prevent thromboembolic complications.

c) Cardioversion:

If an arrhythmia is not resolved with medication, electrical cardioversion (shock) can be performed to restore a normal rhythm.

d) Modulation of Risk Factors:

Correct electrolyte imbalances, control pain to minimise stress, and limit caffeine and other stimulants.

The role of nurses

Nurses play a central role in detecting, managing and educating patients about post-operative arrhythmias. They must be trained to recognise arrhythmias on monitors, to manage antiarrhythmic drugs, and to prepare and assist during cardioversion. In addition, patient education on the recognition of arrhythmia symptoms and the need for prompt intervention is essential.

Post-operative arrhythmias are a major concern after cardiac surgery. Appropriate and proactive management can minimise complications and improve patient outcomes.

Heart failure post-surgical

Post-surgical heart failure is a serious complication that can occur after heart surgery. It is characterised by the inability of the heart to pump enough blood to meet the body's needs. This condition can result from a variety of factors, ranging from direct cardiac injury during surgery to indirect complications. Prompt and effective management of this condition is essential to optimise patient outcomes.

Causes of Post-Surgical Heart Failure
a) Direct myocardial damage:
Manipulation or incision of the heart muscle during surgery may temporarily impair cardiac function.

b) Myocardial ischaemia:
Insufficient oxygen supply to the heart muscle, often due to occlusion or reduced blood flow in the coronary arteries, can lead to heart failure.
c) Post-operative hypertension:
High blood pressure after surgery can increase the workload on the heart, causing or worsening heart failure.

d) Valvular complications:
Problems with the heart valves, whether pre-existing or resulting from surgery, can lead to heart failure.

e) Arrhythmias:
As mentioned above, irregularities in heart rhythm can disrupt the heart's pumping efficiency.

Symptoms and signs
a) Dyspnoea:

Shortness of breath, particularly when exercising or lying down.

b) Oedema:
Swelling, usually of the legs, ankles or feet, caused by an accumulation of fluid.

c) Fatigue:
Weakness or exhaustion can result from an insufficient supply of oxygen to the tissues.

d) Jugular distension:
Swelling of the neck veins may be observed.

e) Lung rales:
Crepitations may be heard when the lungs are auscultated.

Taking charge
a) Medication:
Diuretics to reduce excess fluid, inotropes to strengthen the heart's contraction force, and other drugs to improve heart function may be prescribed.

b) Oxygen therapy:
The administration of supplementary oxygen can help compensate for the lack of oxygen due to poor circulation.

c) Surveillance:
Close monitoring, including echocardiography, electrocardiography and other tests, is essential to assess and adjust treatment.

d) Invasive procedures:
In severe cases, ventricular assist devices or even a heart transplant may be necessary.

The role of nurses
Nurses are on the front line in detecting signs of post-surgical heart failure. They regularly assess the patient's haemodynamic status, administer prescribed medication, monitor side effects and responses to treatment, and educate patients and their families about home care and monitoring. Their vigilance and expertise are essential in optimising care for patients with this complication.

Post-surgical heart failure, although a dreaded complication, is manageable with the right management. Early detection, prompt intervention and close collaboration between doctors, nurses and other healthcare professionals are the key to an optimal outcome.

Complications linked to medical devices (pacemakers, shunts, valves)

Medical devices such as pacemakers, shunts and heart valves have revolutionised the treatment of heart disease. These life-saving interventions have improved and prolonged the lives of millions of patients. However, like any medical intervention, they are not without potential complications. Understanding and monitoring these complications is essential to ensure patient safety.

Pacemakers
a) Infection:
Although rare, infection of the implant site is a serious complication that may require removal of the device and prolonged antibiotic therapy.

b) Moving the probes:

The pacemaker wires can sometimes move from their initial position, requiring repositioning.

c) Discharged batteries:
The pacemaker's batteries have a limited lifespan and need to be replaced periodically.

d) Interference:
Other electronic or medical devices, such as defibrillators or certain medical machines, may interfere with the operation of the pacemaker.

Coronary bypass grafts
a) Graft occlusion:
The leads can become blocked over time, leading to ischaemia or a heart attack.

b) Post-operative bleeding:
All heart surgery can lead to bleeding, which may require intervention.

c) Lung problems:
Pneumonia and fluid accumulation in the lungs are possible complications.

Heart valves
a) Valvular thrombosis:
Blood clots can form on or around the artificial valves, which can obstruct blood flow or cause an embolism.

b) Endocarditis:
Infections can affect valves, particularly artificial ones.

c) Valvular dysfunction:
Valves can deteriorate or fail to function properly, leading to leakage (regurgitation) or narrowing (stenosis).

<u>d) Haemorrhage:</u>
Some patients with mechanical valves require lifelong anticoagulation, which increases the risk of haemorrhage.

Medical technology in cardiology has made enormous strides, offering innovative solutions to previously intractable heart problems. However, it is vital to remain vigilant about possible complications. The involvement of healthcare professionals, and in particular nurses, in the education, monitoring and management of patients fitted with these devices is essential to ensure not only the longevity of these procedures but also the overall well-being of the patient.

Chapter 10:
TOOLS AND TECHNOLOGY
IN CARDIAC SURGERY

Cardiac monitors
and monitoring equipment

Cardiac monitors and monitoring devices are essential tools in cardiology, enabling the electrical and haemodynamic activity of the heart to be observed in real time. They are used in a variety of settings, from post-operative monitoring to intensive care units and outpatient clinics.

Heart monitors
a) Electrocardiogram (ECG):
This is a graphic representation of the heart's electrical activity. It can identify arrhythmias, signs of ischaemia and other cardiac abnormalities.

b) Holter monitors:
These portable devices record the patient's ECG for 24 hours or more. They are often used to detect intermittent arrhythmias.

c) Telemetry monitors:
Used mainly in hospitals, these wireless devices enable patients' ECGs to be monitored remotely, usually from a central station.

Haemodynamic Monitoring Equipment
a) Blood pressure monitors:
They can be non-invasive (cuffs) or invasive (arterial catheters).

b) Pulse oximeters:
These devices measure oxygen saturation in the blood, usually from the finger, earlobe or foot.

c) Echocardiography:
Using ultrasound, this device can visualise heart structures, assess heart function and detect abnormalities.

d) Cardiac catheterisation and intracardiac pressure monitors:
Special catheters, inserted into the heart, can measure the pressure inside the various heart chambers.

Emerging Technologies
a) Portable monitors and wearables:
Devices such as smartwatches and heart patches can now monitor heart rate and other parameters in real time, alerting users to any irregularities.

b) Remote surveillance systems:
Patients can be monitored at home using devices that transmit data in real time to healthcare professionals.

Importance of Surveillance
Cardiac monitoring is crucial not only for detecting abnormalities but also for guiding treatment. Nurses, doctors and other healthcare professionals rely on these devices to make informed decisions about patient management.
What's more, the ability to monitor patients in real time, whether in hospital or at home, offers peace of mind to patients and their families, knowing that anomalies can be detected quickly.

Cardiac monitors and monitoring devices are at the heart of modern cardiology care. As technology continues to evolve, these tools are becoming increasingly sophisticated, offering a better understanding of the heart and facilitating optimal patient management.

The use of ultrasound and Doppler in the operating theatre

Ultrasound and Doppler have gained a significant place in the operating theatre, mainly because of their ability to provide real-time images of internal structures without the use of radiation. These techniques have revolutionised intraoperative management, giving surgeons and anaesthetists a better understanding of the patient's anatomy and physiology.

Ultrasound in the operating theatre
a) Guidance for procedures:
Ultrasound is often used to guide procedures such as the insertion of central venous catheters, the performance of punctures or biopsies, or the precise location of masses or fluids.

b) Cardiac assessment:
Transoesophageal echocardiography (TEE) is commonly used during heart surgery to assess heart function, the presence of air in the heart chambers or to visualise valves.

c) Pulmonary assessment:
Pulmonary ultrasound can help detect abnormalities such as pneumothorax, pleural effusions or pulmonary consolidation.

Doppler in the Operating Room
a) Assessment of blood flow:
Doppler, which measures the movement of red blood cells, can be used to assess blood flow in vessels. This can be

crucial during vascular surgery or to check the viability of a transplanted organ.

b) Detection of stenoses or obstructions:
By measuring the speed of blood flow, Doppler can help locate and quantify narrowings in arteries or veins.

c) Monitoring cerebral perfusion:
Transcranial Doppler is used during certain surgeries to ensure that the brain is properly perfused.

Advantages of ultrasound and Doppler
a) Non-invasive:
These techniques do not require an invasive procedure, thereby reducing the associated risks.

b) No deregistration:
Unlike X-rays or CT scans, ultrasound and Doppler do not use radiation, which is particularly important for lengthy surgeries.

c) Real-time images:
Surgeons and anaesthetists can make decisions based on current information and not on pre-operative images that may no longer be representative of the situation.

The integration of ultrasound and Doppler in the operating theatre has undoubtedly improved the safety and efficiency of surgical procedures. These tools offer a direct window onto the patient's anatomy and physiology, enabling better management and potentially reducing complications. As with any technology, their use requires training and expertise, but the benefits they bring make them invaluable tools for the surgical team.

Recent innovations
and their impact on nursing practice

The world of medicine has witnessed many innovations in recent years. These advances, whether in new technologies or methodologies, have a profound impact on nursing practice, transforming the way care is delivered and improving the quality of care for patients. Let's explore these innovations and their impact on the nursing profession.

Telemedicine and remote care
With the development of communication technologies, telemedicine has become a reality. For nurses :
a) **Remote monitoring:** Portable devices enable continuous monitoring of various physiological parameters, with alerts transmitted in real time to carers.
b) **Virtual consultations:** Nurses can now consult patients remotely, which is particularly useful for remote populations or those with reduced mobility.

Artificial Intelligence (AI) and Data Analysis
a) **Diagnostic assistance:** Sophisticated algorithms can help identify anomalies in patient data, providing valuable support in the diagnostic process.
b) **Case management:** AI systems can automate certain administrative tasks, freeing up time for direct patient care.

Robotics and Automation
a) **Assistance robots:** In some hospitals, robots assist nurses with transporting medicines or equipment, or even with tasks such as disinfection.
b) **Robot-assisted surgery:** Although generally managed by surgeons, this technology requires nurses to be trained in the specifics of robotic assistance, particularly with regard to preparation and maintenance.

<u>Training and Virtual Reality</u>
a) Simulations: Nurses can practise complex procedures in a virtual environment before performing them on real patients.
b) Skills monitoring: Virtual reality systems can assess nurses' skills in real time, enabling continuous improvement.

Innovations in medicines and treatments

Advances in genomics and personalised pharmacology mean that treatments can be tailored to the individual. Nurses play an essential role in monitoring patient responses and managing side effects.

<u>Impact on nursing practice</u>
a) Training requirements: The need for ongoing training to keep up with the latest technologies.
b) Improving the quality of care: Innovations can enable problems to be detected at an early stage and intervention to be more effective.
c) New ethical challenges: Technology raises questions about patient privacy, data security and equitable access to care.

Innovations in medicine and technology have profoundly transformed the nursing profession. While these advances offer many opportunities to improve patient care, they also require nurses to continually adapt, learn new skills and face new challenges. However, at the heart of these changes, the essence of the nursing profession - compassion, empathy and commitment to the well-being of patients - remains unshakeable.

Chapter 11:
PATIENT SAFETY
AND INFECTION PREVENTION

Healthcare-associated infections and their prevention

Healthcare-associated infections (HAIs) are a major concern in healthcare establishments. They occur when a patient becomes infected during the provision of medical care. HCAIs can have serious consequences, ranging from prolonged hospitalisation to permanent sequelae and even death. Understanding their origins and mechanisms is essential if effective preventive measures are to be put in place.

Origins of IAS
Infections can be caused by a variety of micro-organisms, including bacteria, viruses and fungi. In a medical environment :

a) Endogenous flora: Patients naturally carry micro-organisms which, in certain circumstances, can become pathogenic.

b) Cross-transmission: Caregivers may unintentionally transmit micro-organisms from one patient to another.

c) Hospital environment: Surfaces, air and water can be contaminated and become sources of infection.

Common types of IAS
a) Surgical site infections: Occurring after surgery.

b) Catheter-associated infections: In particular, insertion site or bloodstream infections associated with central venous catheters.

c) Ventilation-associated pneumonia: In patients undergoing mechanical ventilation.

d) Urinary tract infections associated with bladder catheterisation.

Prevention of HCAI

a) Hand hygiene: Regular and thorough hand washing is the most effective way of preventing transmission.

b) Wearing personal protective equipment: Gloves, masks, gowns and glasses can protect both the carer and the patient.

c) Aseptic techniques: When carrying out invasive procedures, to ensure a sterile environment.

d) Cleaning and disinfection: Regular cleaning of surfaces and medical equipment.

e) Training and awareness: Regularly inform and train medical staff in good practice.

f) Surveillance and audit: Identify outbreaks of infection quickly and take action.

g) Vaccination: Protecting patients and staff against certain infections.

h) Isolation precautions : For patients infected or colonised by resistant or highly transmissible micro-organisms.

Healthcare-associated infections are a major public health and patient safety issue. Prevention is based on a combination of simple and complex measures involving all medical staff. Thanks to constant vigilance, ongoing training and a culture of safety, it is possible to significantly reduce the risk of HCAI and guarantee better quality of care for all patients.

Asepsis and sterilisation protocols in cardiac surgery

Asepsis and sterilisation in cardiac surgery are crucial to preventing post-operative infections. A rigorous protocol is essential to guarantee patient safety. The integrity of these protocols guarantees contamination-free surgery.

Asepsis protocol

a) Hand washing: Thorough hand washing, lasting 2 to 6 minutes, using a surgical technique with a special brush and a suitable antiseptic, is the first step.

b) Wearing sterile garments: Surgical garments, consisting of a gown, mask, cap and sterile gloves, are essential. Double gloving is recommended for high-risk procedures.

c) Preparing the patient : The surgical area is shaved (if necessary) and then cleaned with an antiseptic solution, often iodine- or chlorhexidine-based.

d) Use of sterile drapes: These are placed around the operating area to create a sterile space.

e) Aseptic handling: Any material or instrument entering the sterile field must be handled aseptically.

Sterilisation protocol

a) Pre-cleaning: Before sterilisation, instruments must be thoroughly cleaned. Instruments are soaked and brushed to remove any residue.

b) Autoclaving: Surgical instruments are placed in an autoclave which uses pressurised steam to kill micro-organisms.

c) Ethylene oxide gas: For instruments that cannot be autoclaved, such as certain electronic or plastic components.

d) Sterility check: After sterilisation, a check is carried out, generally using chemical or biological indicators, to ensure that the process has been effective.

e) Storage: Sterilised instruments should be stored in a clean, dry, dust-free place.

f) Post-sterilisation handling: Sterilised instruments are handled with care to avoid contamination before use.

Special features of cardiac surgery

In cardiac surgery, certain items of equipment, such as cannulas, circulatory support circuits or pacemakers, require special attention when it comes to sterilisation. What's more, given the complexity of certain procedures, the surgical team must ensure that every member is well informed and trained in asepsis and sterilisation protocols.

Scrupulous compliance with asepsis and sterilisation protocols in cardiac surgery is vital. The slightest failure can lead to serious complications for the patient. Each member of the surgical team has a decisive role to play in guaranteeing the safety and success of the operation.

Managing situations contamination or medical errors

Managing situations involving contamination or medical errors is a major challenge for healthcare establishments. Although rare, these events can have dramatic consequences for patients and lead to a loss of confidence in the healthcare system. A systematic, transparent and caring approach is essential to managing these situations.

<u>Recognition and assessment</u>

a) Rapid identification: As soon as contamination or an error is suspected or identified, it is crucial to inform the medical team concerned.

b) Clinical assessment of the patient : The patient must be assessed immediately to determine the seriousness of the situation and the necessary interventions.

Communication

a) Informing the patient: It is imperative to inform the patient or their family in a transparent, honest and empathetic way, explaining what has happened, the implications and the next steps.

b) Internal reporting : Medical errors and contamination must be reported using the facility's internal systems to ensure traceability and subsequent analysis.

Medical intervention

a) Immediate treatment: Depending on the nature of the error or contamination, medical interventions may be necessary to stabilise the patient or prevent complications.

b) Follow-up: Patients must receive regular follow-up to detect and manage any after-effects.

Analysis of the event

a) Analysis meeting: A team meeting is organised to understand the chain of events that led to the error or contamination.

b) Systemic approach: Errors are generally the result of a series of systemic failures and not the fault of an individual. It is essential to adopt a systemic approach to identify the root causes.

Corrective measures

a) Procedural improvements: Based on the analysis of the event, changes to protocols and procedures may be necessary to prevent the error from recurring.

b) Training: Teams may require additional training to avoid similar mistakes in the future.

<u>Psychological support</u>
a) For the patient : Experiencing a medical error or contamination can be traumatic. Psychological support must be offered to patients and their families.
b) For the medical team: The carers involved may feel guilty, stressed or anxious. They must also be given psychological support and a forum for discussion.

Managing situations of contamination or medical errors requires a multidimensional response, centred on the patient but also attentive to the well-being of the medical team. Transparency, empathy and a commitment to continuous improvement in healthcare systems are essential to restoring trust and ensuring patient safety in the future.

Chapter 12:
PHARMACOLOGY
IN CARDIAC SURGERY

Cardiotropic drugs
and their administration

Cardiotropic drugs are an essential class of medicines in cardiology. They act specifically on the heart and blood vessels to treat various heart conditions, improving patients' quality of life and, in many cases, increasing their life expectancy.
Introduction to cardiotropic drugs

Cardiotropic medicines are essentially designed to influence cardiac function. Whether they are used to regulate heart rate, increase or decrease the force of contraction, or influence blood pressure, these drugs play a fundamental role in the management of heart disease.

Categorisation of cardiotropic medicines
Inotropes: These drugs influence the contraction force of the heart muscle.
Examples: digoxin, dobutamine.
Chronotropics: These act on the heart rate.
Examples: atropine (positive), propranolol (negative).
Dromotropes: These drugs affect the speed of electrical conduction in the heart.
Examples: beta-blockers, verapamil.
Vasodilators: They dilate blood vessels, reducing peripheral resistance and blood pressure.
Examples: nitrates, diltiazem.

Diuretics: They increase urine production, helping to reduce the heart's workload by reducing the volume of blood.

Examples: furosemide, hydrochlorothiazide.

Administration and supervision

The administration of cardiotropic drugs requires special attention and regular monitoring because of their direct impact on cardiac function.

Dosage: It is crucial to administer the correct dose, as an underdose can be ineffective, while an overdose can cause serious side effects.

Routes of administration: Some drugs are administered orally, others intravenously, and still others by more specialised methods. The route of administration is chosen according to the patient's condition and the speed of action required.

Monitoring: Vital signs, in particular blood pressure, heart rate and respiratory rate, should be monitored regularly. Blood tests may also be necessary to monitor drug levels or detect possible side effects.

Drug interactions: Many cardiotropic drugs can interact with other drugs, requiring careful prescription management and monitoring.

Cardiotropic drugs are indispensable tools in the treatment of heart disease. However, their effectiveness depends on proper administration, rigorous monitoring and a thorough understanding of their mechanism of action and potential interactions.

Interaction and monitoring side effects

Drug interaction and the monitoring of side effects are key factors in the management of patients undergoing cardiotropic treatment, and more generally, any medical treatment. The ability to anticipate, identify and manage these factors can not only optimise treatment efficacy but also prevent potentially serious complications.

Drug interactions
Drug interactions occur when the effect of one drug is altered by taking another drug, food, drink or substance. They may potentiate or diminish the therapeutic effect, or give rise to new undesirable effects.

- Types of interactions :
  - **Synergistic:** Two drugs act together to produce a stronger or additional effect.
  - **Antagonists:** One drug reduces the effectiveness of the other.
  - **Metabolic changes:** Some medicines can influence the way other medicines are metabolised in the body.
- Prevention :
  - It is vital to know about all the medicines and food supplements the patient is taking.
  - Drug databases and modern IT tools can help to identify potential interactions.
- Management :
  - If an interaction is identified, the dose may need to be adjusted or the drug changed.
  - Close clinical monitoring is often required to ensure that the patient remains stable.

Monitoring side effects
Every drug has the potential to cause side effects, some minor, others more serious.
- Identification :
  - Open communication with the patient is essential. They should be encouraged to report any unusual symptoms.

- Regular check-ups, particularly blood tests, may be necessary for certain medicines, in order to identify abnormalities before they become a problem.

Management :
- If a side effect is identified, its seriousness needs to be assessed. In some cases, simple monitoring will suffice; in others, treatment adjustment or hospitalisation may be required.
- Patient education is essential. They must be informed of the potential side-effects of their medication and what to do if they occur.

Drug interactions and side effects can present challenges to medical management, but with appropriate monitoring, effective communication and sound patient education, these challenges can be overcome, ensuring the best possible patient care.

Anticoagulants and antithrombotics: management and monitoring

Anticoagulants and antithrombotics are essential medicines for preventing and treating the formation of blood clots in blood vessels or the heart. Their use requires particular attention and rigorous monitoring, as excessive or insufficient anticoagulation can lead to serious complications.

Anticoagulants and antithrombotics: an overview
- **Objective:** The aim of these drugs is to reduce the risk of thrombus formation (blood clots), which can lead to strokes, heart attacks or embolisms.
- Main agents :
  - **Anticoagulants :** Heparin, Warfarin, Dabigatran, Rivaroxaban.

Antiplatelet agents (subclass of antithrombotics) : Aspirin, Clopidogrel, Prasugrel.

Managing anticoagulants and antithrombotics

Determining the dose: The dose should be adjusted according to the patient's condition, the pathology to be treated, and other factors such as weight and age.

Duration of treatment: Some patients will require treatment for life, while others will only need it for a limited period.

Regular monitoring: For patients taking Warfarin, for example, the prothrombin time (INR) should be checked regularly to ensure that the level of anticoagulation is adequate.

Monitoring side effects

Bleeding: This is the most common side effect. Patients should be made aware of signs to watch for, such as unusual bruising, blood in the urine or stools, or prolonged bleeding after an injury.

Drug interactions: Many drugs can interact with anticoagulants, increasing or decreasing their efficacy. It is essential to keep all associated treatments up to date.

Other side effects: Some patients may experience allergic reactions, liver problems or other symptoms. It is essential to report any unusual symptoms to your doctor.

Patient education

Signs of bleeding: It is essential to inform patients of the risks of bleeding and the signs to watch out for.

Regular monitoring: Patients need to understand the importance of regular checks, such as blood tests to monitor the efficacy and safety of treatment.

Lifestyle: It may be necessary to give recommendations on diet, physical activity and other aspects of lifestyle to minimise the risks.

The management and monitoring of anticoagulants and antithrombotics are crucial to optimising their benefits while minimising the associated risks. Transparent communication between the healthcare professional and the patient, together with appropriate education, are the keys to successful therapy.

Chapter 13:
PAIN MANAGEMENT
IN CARDIAC SURGERY

Pain assessment and scales

Assessing pain is a fundamental step in the clinical management of any patient. Pain, often referred to as the "fifth vital sign", is subjective and unique to each individual. Yet quantifying it is essential in order to personalise and adjust treatment. Numerous scales have been developed to assess this sensory and emotional experience as objectively as possible.

The importance of pain assessment
Pain assessment enables :
- Understand the intensity and nature of the pain experienced by the patient.
- Adapt and guide the therapeutic plan.
- Monitor the progress of pain and the effectiveness of interventions.

Pain assessment scales
- **Visual Analogue Scale (VAS): This is a** 10 cm ruler with no numbers, ranging from "no pain" to "unbearable pain". Patients mark the intensity of their pain on the scale.
- **Numerical Scale (EN):** Patients are asked to quantify their pain on a scale ranging from 0 (no pain) to 10 (maximum imaginable pain).
- **Simple Verbal Scale (EVS):** The patient describes their level of pain using predefined terms such as "none", "mild", "moderate" or "severe".
- **Pain scale for children :** Children may have difficulty using traditional scales. The face scale (such

as the Wong-Baker scale) allows children to select a face corresponding to their level of pain.

Scales for non-communicative people: For patients who cannot express themselves (newborn babies, certain elderly patients, patients with neurological conditions, etc.), other scales have been developed. These scales, such as the FLACC scale (Face, Legs, Activity, Cry, Consolability), assess pain by observing the patient's behaviour and reactions.

Other assessment considerations

Nature and location: It is essential to understand the type of pain (dull, stabbing, burning, etc.) and its location in order to guide the diagnosis and treatment.

Triggering or aggravating factors: Understanding what increases or decreases pain can help to adjust treatment.

Impact on daily life: How does pain affect sleep, appetite, mood, or the ability to carry out daily activities?

Pain assessment is a pivotal element in holistic patient management. By using appropriate scales and learning more about the patient's experience of pain, carers can personalise interventions and maximise patient comfort and well-being.

Pharmacological techniques and non-pharmacological

Pain management, whether acute or chronic, relies on a wide range of methods, both pharmacological and non-pharmacological. These methods can be used alone or in combination to provide optimal pain management tailored to the individual patient.

Pharmacological techniques

Non-opioid analgesics: These drugs, such as paracetamol and non-steroidal anti-inflammatory drugs (NSAIDs), are used to treat mild to moderate pain.

Opioids: Used to treat moderate to severe pain, these drugs include morphine, codeine and oxycodone, among others.

Local anaesthetics: These temporarily block sensation in a specific part of the body. Examples include lidocaine and bupivacaine.

Co-analgesics or adjuvants: These are drugs which are not primarily designed as analgesics but which have analgesic properties under certain conditions. These include certain anticonvulsants, antidepressants and muscle relaxants.

Corticosteroids: These can be used to reduce inflammation and pain, particularly in cases of joint or nerve inflammation.

Non-pharmacological techniques

Physical therapy: Modalities such as heat, cold, massage, ultrasound therapy and transcutaneous electrical nerve stimulation (TENS) can help relieve pain.

Exercise: Appropriate, targeted movements can reduce pain, improve mobility and strengthen muscles.

Acupuncture: This ancient Chinese technique uses fine needles inserted at specific points to balance energy flows and reduce pain.

Biofeedback: This is a technique in which the patient learns to control certain physiological functions to improve pain.

Cognitive behavioural therapy (CBT): This therapeutic approach helps patients to recognise and change the negative thought patterns associated with their pain.

Meditation and relaxation: These techniques help to reduce stress and tension, which can exacerbate pain.

Distraction techniques: Concentrating on a positive activity or thought can divert attention from the pain.

Touch therapy: Like massage or reflexology, it can relax and relieve tension.

Pain management is an essential aspect of patient care. By combining pharmacological and non-pharmacological techniques, healthcare professionals can offer a more holistic and individualised approach to pain management, taking into account both the physical and emotional well-being of the patient.

Chronic post-surgical pain: recognition and management

Chronic post-surgical pain is a problem that affects a significant proportion of patients following surgery. Its persistence beyond the expected recovery period represents a challenge for both the patient and the healthcare team. Recognising and managing this pain is crucial to the patient's well-being and recovery.

Recognition of Chronic Post-Surgical Pain

1. Definition: Chronic post-surgical pain is pain that persists for more than three months after surgery, without any other apparent cause.

2. Signs and symptoms: It may manifest itself as continuous or intermittent pain, hypersensitivity of the operated area, exacerbated pain on touching or impairment of normal functions.

3. Assessment: Regular pain assessment using standardised scales and questionnaires helps to identify and quantify pain.

Risk Factors
1. Type of surgery: Some procedures, such as thoracic surgery, are more likely to result in chronic post-operative pain.
2. Pain history: Patients who have suffered chronic pain before the operation or who have experienced intense acute pain after the operation are at greater risk.
3. Psychological factors: Anxiety, depression or low resilience to pain can increase the risk of chronic pain.

Taking charge
1. Pharmacological approach: Analgesics, including opioids, NSAIDs, anticonvulsants and antidepressants, may be used. Prescription must be tailored to the individual patient.
2. Physical therapies: Physiotherapy, exercises, TENS and other modalities can help manage pain.
3. Interventional interventions: Nerve blocks, injections or even surgery may be considered to treat the underlying cause.
4. Psychological approach: CBT, relaxation and other therapies can help manage the stress, anxiety and depression associated with pain.
5. Complementary approaches: Acupuncture, massage and meditation can also be beneficial.

Education and monitoring
It is crucial to educate patients about post-surgical pain, risk factors and management methods. Regular monitoring allows treatments to be adjusted and any complications or new causes of pain to be identified quickly.

Chronic post-surgical pain is a medical challenge that requires a multidisciplinary approach. Early management, recognition of risk factors, appropriate education and rigorous follow-up are essential to ensure the best possible quality of life for the patient.

Chapter 14:
INTERNATIONAL
AND CARDIAC SURGERY

Taking part in missions
or abroad

Taking part in humanitarian missions or working abroad is an experience that offers nurses a unique and enriching perspective. By working in contexts different from their usual environment, nurses not only acquire new skills, but also develop a deeper understanding of global health challenges.

The reasons behind these missions

Altruistic commitment: Many are driven by a desire to help vulnerable populations, to provide care where it is most needed, and to make a tangible difference to people's lives.

Acquiring skills: These missions offer the opportunity to develop new clinical skills, to learn how to manage rare diseases or diseases specific to certain regions, and to work in sometimes precarious conditions.

Cultural enrichment: Working abroad or on a humanitarian mission allows you to immerse yourself in a new culture, understand other ways of life and broaden your horizons.

Preparation and planning

Research and selection: It is essential to find an organisation or programme that matches your values and skills. Some focus on emergency care, while others may concentrate on community health or education.

Training: Nurses may need specific training before they leave, such as courses on tropical diseases, travel medicine or international health.

Logistical considerations: Vaccinations, visas, accommodation and other practicalities need to be taken into account.

Challenges and rewards

Limited resources: Working in remote areas or in humanitarian contexts can mean having to cope with a lack of equipment, medicines or personnel.

Language and cultural barriers: Communication can be a challenge, making it essential to respect and understand the local culture.

Emotional resilience: Nurses can be faced with heartbreaking situations, requiring mental strength and adequate support.

Positive impact: Despite the challenges, many nurses return from these missions with a renewed appreciation for their profession, lasting memories, and the satisfaction of having made a positive difference.

Future prospects

- Taking part in humanitarian or overseas missions can also open doors to leadership roles, specialisations or further training opportunities. It's an experience that, although sometimes trying, is often described as invaluable by those who choose to take this path.

Whether it's a desire to help, a need for adventure, or a combination of both, taking part in humanitarian missions or working abroad offers nurses a unique opportunity to broaden their professional and personal horizons. By enriching the mind and spirit, these experiences often redefine the way nurses perceive and practise their profession.

Differences in practice
and ethics on the international stage

Cardiac surgery, like other medical disciplines, can vary considerably from one part of the world to another, not only in terms of practice but also in terms of ethics. When talking about international differences, it is essential to recognise that these variations can be influenced by a mixture of cultural, economic, political and social factors.

Differences in practice

- **Techniques and procedures:** The surgical techniques adopted may vary according to the training available, medical traditions and accessible technologies.
- **Access to resources:** In developing countries, access to state-of-the-art equipment and medicines can be limited, which influences the way care is delivered.
- **Training and specialisation:** Training and specialisation pathways can differ considerably, with countries emphasising different skills and areas of knowledge.
- **Roles of healthcare professionals:** In some cultures, nurses may have more extensive or more limited roles, depending on their training and local traditions.

Ethical differences

- **Informed consent:** Although the concept of informed consent is universal, the way in which it is obtained and valued can vary. In some cultures, it may be common practice to consult the family before making medical decisions, while in others, patient autonomy is paramount.

- **End-of-life issues:** Decisions about resuscitation, stopping treatment or palliative care may be influenced by religious or cultural beliefs.
- **Confidentiality:** Expectations of confidentiality and information sharing may vary, particularly in cultures where families play a more central role in patient care.
- **Priorities in care:** In certain contexts, where resources are limited, difficult decisions can be made about who receives treatment on the basis of criteria other than purely medical ones, such as age or social status.

Navigating the differences

For healthcare professionals working internationally or collaborating with colleagues in other countries, it is crucial to :

- **Be informed:** Understand local contexts, medical practices and ethical nuances.
- **Listen:** Be open to the views and experiences of others, recognising that there is not always one 'right' way of doing things.
- **Collaborate:** Working together to share knowledge, respect different approaches and find solutions that focus on the patient's well-being.

International differences in practice and ethics reflect the diversity and complexity of the world in which we live. By understanding and respecting these differences, healthcare professionals can provide more compassionate, effective and responsive care to patients around the world.

International exchanges and collaborations to enhance your practice

The world of healthcare is characterised by constant innovation and change, and this is especially true in the field of cardiac surgery, where new techniques and technologies regularly emerge. Cardiac surgery nurses, in addition to their essential role with patients, can greatly benefit from international exchanges and collaboration to enrich their practice.

Professional exchanges
- Exchange programmes :
- International exchange programmes offer nurses the opportunity to learn new methods and approaches by working in a variety of contexts.
- They allow immersion in other healthcare cultures, contributing to a deeper understanding of global healthcare.
- Conferences and Seminars :
- Taking part in international conferences not only enables you to acquire new knowledge, but also to forge links with professionals from all over the world.
- Seminars and workshops provide opportunities for continuing education and skills development.

Research collaborations
- Joint research projects :
- International collaboration can encourage joint research projects, enabling the exchange of data and research results.
- Collaborative research increases the scope and impact of studies, contributing to the overall advancement of the discipline.
- Publications :
- By publishing articles in international journals, you can share your own experience and research with a wider audience.
- Reading international publications offers different perspectives and up-to-date information on advances in the field.

Collaboration for Training and Education

Sharing educational resources :
International collaboration offers the opportunity to share and access educational resources such as e-learning modules, case studies and course materials.

Mentoring programmes :
International mentoring programmes enable nurses to benefit from the experience and advice of experienced professionals from all over the world.

Development of Protocols and Guidelines

Joint development of protocols :
Working with international colleagues to develop protocols and clinical guidelines can help ensure that care is at the forefront of global practice.

In an increasingly interconnected world, opportunities for international exchange and collaboration are not only accessible, but essential to enriching the practice of cardiac surgery nurses. They offer opportunities to learn, share knowledge and skills, and ultimately contribute to improving patient care worldwide.

Chapter 15:
NUTRITION AND FOOD HYGIENE IN CARDIAC PATIENTS

The importance of nutrition in recovery and prevention

Nutrition plays a crucial role in heart health, both for those who have already undergone heart surgery and for those seeking to prevent heart disease. The relationship between nutrition, post-operative recovery and the prevention of heart disease is intimate and complex, reflecting the way in which our diet influences every facet of our well-being.

Nutrition and Post-Operative Recovery
   Healing wounds :
      After surgery, the body requires specific nutrients to help repair tissues. Quality proteins, vitamins such as vitamin C and minerals such as zinc are essential for optimal healing.
   Energy and strength :
      Post-surgical recovery can be exhausting. A nutrient-rich diet provides the energy needed to help patients regain their strength and stamina.
   Immune function :
      The good fats, proteins, vitamins and minerals help to strengthen the immune system, reducing the risk of post-operative infections.
Nutrition and prevention of heart disease
   Cholesterol reduction :
      A diet low in saturated and trans f a t s , combined with fibre-rich foods, can help

reduce blood cholesterol, a major risk factor for heart disease.

Blood Pressure Control :
  Diets rich in fruit, vegetables, whole grains and low sodium help to maintain healthy blood pressure, thereby protecting the heart.

Weight management :
  Maintaining a healthy weight is crucial for heart health. Balanced nutrition, combined with regular physical activity, can help achieve and maintain an optimal weight.

Reduced inflammation :
  Certain foods, such as those rich in omega-3, have natural anti-inflammatory properties that can help reduce the risk of heart disease.

Specific Nutrition for Heart Patients

Sodium control :
  For patients suffering from heart failure or hypertension, it is particularly important to monitor sodium intake to avoid fluid overload and excessive blood pressure.

Antioxidants and Phytonutrients :
  Fruit, vegetables and other plant sources are rich in antioxidants and phytonutrients that protect the heart from oxidative damage.

Nutrition is a fundamental pillar of heart health. Whether to promote rapid and complete recovery after surgery or to prevent heart disease, a healthy, balanced diet is an investment in long-term health. For heart patients, working closely with dieticians and health professionals can help to develop a nutritional plan tailored to their specific needs.

Specific dietary advice
for cardiac patients

Nutrition plays a vital role in the management and prevention of heart disease. Dietary choices can influence many risk factors, such as cholesterol, blood pressure, inflammation and obesity. For heart patients, adopting a cardio-healthy diet is essential. Here are a few recommendations to guide these patients.

Limit salt :
Reduce your salt intake to help manage hypertension. Favour homemade foods and limit processed foods, which are often high in sodium.

Eat healthy fats:
Opt for the unsaturated fats found in olive, canola and sunflower oils. Include sources of omega-3, such as salmon, flaxseed and walnuts. Limit saturated fats and avoid trans fats.

Add more fruit and vegetables:
Rich in vitamins, minerals and fibre, fruit and vegetables help to reduce blood pressure and protect against atherosclerosis.

Go for lean proteins:
Choose lean meats, skinless poultry, fish and vegetarian alternatives such as pulses and tofu.

Add wholegrain cereals:
Foods such as oats, quinoa, brown rice and wholemeal bread provide heart-healthy fibre.

Reduce Alcohol Consumption:
If you drink, do so in moderation. Alcohol can increase blood pressure.

- Limit Added Sugar :
    - Sugary drinks, pastries and other foods rich in added sugars can contribute to weight gain and increase the risk of heart disease.
- Watch your weight:
    - Maintaining a healthy weight is crucial for heart health. A balanced diet, combined with regular exercise, will help you achieve this goal.
- Stay hydrated:
    - Drinking enough water is essential for your body and heart to function at their best.
- Read the Tags :
    - Learning to read nutrition labels can help you make healthier food choices. Pay attention to sodium levels, types of fat and added sugars.
- Consult a Nutritionist:
    - For personalised advice, consult a dietician-nutritionist who will be able to help you draw up a meal plan tailored to your needs.

By adopting this advice and gradually modifying their diet, heart patients can positively influence their heart health, improve their quality of life and reduce the risk of future complications. Adopting a cardiosan diet is a long-term commitment, but it is a worthwhile investment in health.

Working with dieticians for suitable food plans

At the heart of multidisciplinary medical teams lies an essential but sometimes underestimated collaboration: that between the nurse and the dietician. Their alliance is crucial to ensuring the best possible patient care, especially in areas where nutrition plays a key role, such as cardiac surgery.

As soon as a patient arrives, the nurse, in his or her central role as carer, collects data on the patient's general condition, eating habits, any allergies or culinary preferences. This information, once relayed to the dietician, enables an initial nutritional diagnosis to be made and a suitable dietary strategy to be defined.

The dietician, with his in-depth knowledge of nutrition, will then draw up a tailor-made diet plan. This plan will take into account the patient's specific needs, whether to prepare the body for surgery, to promote optimal recovery or to manage co-morbidities such as diabetes. The nurse, by virtue of his or her proximity to the patient, plays a pivotal role in monitoring this plan, observing the patient's reaction to the meals served and gathering feedback.

But beyond this technical management, this collaboration has a human dimension. Meals become key moments in a hospitalised patient's day. They punctuate the day, provide comfort, and can even be indicators of morale and motivation. The nurse, through his or her daily presence, and the dietician, through his or her expertise, work together to make these moments moments of well-being, listening and appropriate care.

The success of this collaboration also lies in communication and ongoing training. Advances in nutrition are constant, and it is vital that nurses and dieticians share their knowledge, discuss complex cases and learn about new recommendations together.

By combining their strengths, expertise and humanity, nurses and dieticians can guarantee comprehensive, patient-centred nutritional care, making a major contribution to improving patients' health and quality of life.

Chapter 16:
Cardiac rehabilitation

Principles and objectives cardiac rehabilitation

Cardiac rehabilitation is a medically supervised process designed to improve the health and well-being of people with heart problems or who have undergone cardiac surgery. It is based on a holistic approach, combining physical training, therapeutic education and psychosocial support to help patients regain an optimal quality of life.

The fundamental principles of cardiac rehabilitation are:

- **Personalisation**: Each programme is tailored to the patient's specific needs, taking into account their physical capabilities, medical history and personal goals.
- **Multidisciplinarity**: Cardiac rehabilitation is the result of collaboration between cardiologists, physiotherapists, nurses, dieticians, psychologists and other specialists to provide comprehensive care.
- **Continuity of care**: Rehabilitation often extends over several weeks or months, requiring regular monitoring and periodic assessment of progress.
- **Holistic approach**: Beyond the physical aspect, rehabilitation also encompasses psychological, nutritional and social aspects to treat the patient as a whole.

The main objectives of cardiac rehabilitation are :

- **Improved physical capacity**: Through progressive exercises, patients strengthen their heart, improve their endurance and muscular strength.

Optimising risk factors: Rehabilitation aims to help patients control and reduce the risk factors associated with heart disease, such as high blood pressure, high cholesterol, obesity or smoking.

Therapeutic education: Patients learn to better understand their disease, the medication they are taking and the lifestyle changes needed to prevent recurrence or progression of their condition.

Psychological support: Heart disease can be traumatic, leading to stress, depression or anxiety. Rehabilitation offers emotional support, helping patients to overcome these psychological challenges.

Social integration: By regaining confidence in themselves and their abilities, patients are encouraged to resume an active social and professional life.

Secondary prevention: One of the key objectives is to prevent new cardiac events by establishing good lifestyle habits and ensuring appropriate medical follow-up.

Cardiac rehabilitation is much more than a simple exercise programme. It is a comprehensive, patient-centred approach designed to give patients back the keys to a full and active life, despite their heart disease.

The role of the nurse in monitoring and support

Nurses play a pivotal role in the care of cardiac patients, often considered to be the essential link between the patient and the medical team. Their unique position, both close to the patient and in close contact with the nursing team, gives them crucial responsibilities in terms of monitoring and support.

Therapeutic education: Nurses are generally the patient's first point of contact for answering questions about their illness, the procedures they have undergone, the medicines they have been prescribed and the lifestyle changes they recommend. They play an active role in patient education, helping patients to better understand their disease and the associated care.

Ongoing assessment: In addition to technical care, nurses carry out regular assessments of the patient's state of health, monitoring key indicators such as vital signs, pain levels and the effectiveness of treatments administered.

Emotional support: Recognising the psychological challenges that heart disease can present, nurses provide attentive listening and constant emotional support. They often witness the patient's anxieties, hopes and concerns, and strive to provide reassuring and caring responses.

Coordinating care: Nurses ensure smooth coordination between the various care providers - doctors, physiotherapists, dieticians, psychologists. They ensure that all care is provided in a harmonious manner, taking into account the specific needs of each patient.

Follow-up at home: After discharge from hospital, the nurse may also be involved in follow-up at home, ensuring that care continues, that medical prescriptions are followed and that any signs of complications are detected early.

Health promotion: Nurses encourage patients to adopt a healthy lifestyle, whether in terms of diet, physical activity, smoking cessation or stress management. They play an active role in secondary prevention, aimed at avoiding recurrences or complications.

Discussions with families: Aware of the impact of the disease on those around them, nurses also provide support to families, guiding them, reassuring them and involving them in the care process.

Nurses are the guarantors of holistic, patient-centred care, combining technical skills, interpersonal know-how and clinical expertise. Their constant presence, attentiveness and dedication make them an essential pillar in the monitoring and support of cardiac patients.

Exercise, returning to work and long-term monitoring

Cardiac surgery, however sophisticated, is just one stage in a heart patient's journey to recovery. The post-operative period is just as crucial, particularly in terms of resuming physical activity, appropriate exercise and long-term monitoring to ensure a return to a healthy life and avoid complications.

Resuming daily activities: After an operation, patients are often anxious about returning to their previous life. This is where the role of the nurse and the rehabilitation team is crucial. They help patients to gradually resume their activities, ranging from simple everyday tasks such as dressing or walking, to more complex activities.

The importance of exercise: Cardiovascular exercises, tailored to each patient, are essential to strengthen the heart and improve endurance and lung capacity. With the support of a physiotherapist, patients are introduced to a series of exercises adapted to their condition, enabling them to resume physical activity gently.

Returning to work and social life: Depending on the nature of their profession, some patients will be able to return to work quickly, while others will need more time to adapt. The nurse helps to determine the right time to return to work and advises on any adjustments that need to be made to the workstation. Similarly, resuming a fulfilling social life is a crucial aspect of rehabilitation.

Long-term medical monitoring: Beyond the first few weeks post-operatively, regular medical monitoring is necessary. This is to ensure that the heart is functioning properly, that the prescribed medication is well tolerated and that the patient is following the lifestyle recommendations. Regular appointments with the cardiologist and other specialists, as well as periodic check-ups, are an integral part of this monitoring.

Education and prevention: Throughout the treatment process, nurses play a key role in patient education. They provide information on warning signs, the benefits of a balanced diet, the importance of giving up smoking and stress management techniques.

Psychological support: Cardiac surgery can leave its mark, and not just physically. Many patients express fears, anxieties or depression. Psychological support, either from a nurse or a psychologist, is essential to overcome these feelings.

The post-operative period in cardiac surgery is a winding road, punctuated by challenges but also victories. Resumption of activity, appropriate exercise and long-term monitoring are key stages in ensuring that patients regain their quality of life, under the kind and expert eye of their nurse.

Chapter 17:
PALLIATIVE CARE IN CARDIOLOGY

Introduction to palliative care in cardiology

Cardiology, although strongly focused on curative interventions and advanced medical solutions, inevitably encounters situations where cure is no longer a viable option. It is at these delicate and trying moments that palliative care takes on its full meaning.

The nature of palliative care: Contrary to common perception, palliative care is not just about "accompanying death". It is a holistic approach aimed at offering patients and their families a better quality of life in the face of a life-threatening illness. This includes managing pain and symptoms, as well as psychological, social and spiritual needs.

Relevance in cardiology: In cardiology, particularly in the case of advanced diseases such as end-stage heart failure, the curative approach can reach its limits. In such cases, it is essential to consider a transition to care that focuses on patient comfort, alleviating symptoms and supporting the patient's family. This care is essential to ensure a dignified and peaceful end to life.

Particular challenges in cardiology: Cardiac diseases present specific challenges for palliative care. Unlike other diseases where progression is relatively predictable, heart disease can progress abruptly and suddenly. This makes care planning, discussions about advance directives and ethical decision-making all the more complex.

The role of the nurse: Nurses play a pivotal role in the implementation of palliative care in cardiology. They are often the first point of contact between the patient, their family and the medical team. Their ability to assess symptoms, communicate effectively, provide emotional support and coordinate with other healthcare professionals is essential to providing quality palliative care.

Communication and Ethics: An important part of palliative care is open and honest communication. Nurses are often called upon to facilitate these delicate discussions about expectations, hopes, fears and decisions concerning the end of life.

A link with the family: Palliative care is not just about the patient. Relatives are also going through an extremely difficult period and need support, information and guidance. The nurse, through his or her proximity and expertise, is a pillar of support for these families.

Palliative care in cardiology is an essential component of overall patient management. It is a reminder that, sometimes, comfort, dignity and humanity prevail over cure. Nurses play a key role in this process, providing both technical expertise and human warmth.

Symptom management and emotional support

Cardiac surgery goes to the very heart of what keeps us alive. Patients confronted with this reality often experience an avalanche of emotions, combined with a variety of physical symptoms that require appropriate management. The key is to manage the symptoms effectively while providing solid emotional support.

The Duality of Symptoms: After cardiac surgery, patients may experience a range of symptoms. These may be physiological, such as pain, fatigue, breathing difficulties or arrhythmias, or psychological, such as anxiety, depression or feelings of vulnerability.

Holistic assessment: A holistic approach is essential to effective care. The nurse must assess both physical and emotional symptoms. Pain assessment scales, mental health questionnaires and regular interviews are valuable tools in this process.

Analgesic strategies: Pain is one of the most common and dreaded symptoms. Nurses must be able to administer the prescribed medication while monitoring for any side effects. At the same time, non-pharmacological techniques such as relaxation or distraction can be effective.

Emotional support: Feelings of anxiety and uncertainty are common after heart surgery. The nurse plays a crucial role in listening and reassuring patients. They are often the health professional closest to the patient, offering not only care but also an attentive ear and a reassuring presence.

Benevolent Communication : The way in which information is conveyed to patients can greatly influence their emotional state. Clear, honest and empathetic communication is fundamental. It's about answering questions, dispelling myths and reinforcing the patient's sense of security.

Family support: The family often plays a key role in the patient's emotional recovery. The nurse must also support, educate and reassure them. Providing them with information, involving them in care and responding to their concerns fosters an environment conducive to recovery.

Referral and collaboration: In more complex cases, nurses may need to work closely with other specialists, such as psychologists, psychiatrists or social workers. Prompt referral can often make the difference in managing symptoms and emotional well-being.

Symptom management and emotional support go hand in hand. Post-operative care is not just about physical healing; it also encompasses emotional and psychological healing. Nurses, through their training and experience, are on the front line in ensuring this delicate balance.

Working in a team
with palliative care specialists

Cardiology, like other medical specialities, is confronted with times when, despite the best possible interventions, a patient's prognosis remains bleak. In these delicate situations, palliative care becomes essential to ensure the patient's quality of life is as good as possible. Cardiac surgery nurses work closely with a team of specialists dedicated to this care. This interdisciplinary relationship is both complex and rewarding, requiring fluid communication, empathy and mutual respect.

Understanding the aims of palliative care : The essence of palliative care is the relief of suffering, whether physical, psychological, social or spiritual. It is not necessarily about the end of life, but about quality of life. Nurses must understand and respect this approach, which focuses on the patient rather than the illness.

The Central Role of Communication: Palliative care teams are often made up of doctors, nurses, social workers, psychologists, chaplains and sometimes other professionals. Coordinating care requires regular and transparent exchanges between all these players to ensure holistic care.

Managing complex symptoms: Palliative care patients may present with a variety of symptoms, ranging from pain to breathlessness or anxiety. Working with a specialist team enables targeted and effective therapeutic strategies to be implemented, enriching the skills of the cardiology nurse.

Emotional and Psychological Support: Nurses are often the first point of contact for patients and their families. Working with palliative care specialists, they can ensure that their emotional needs are recognised and addressed, whether through simple conversation or more structured therapy.

Difficult decisions: Questions may arise about limiting or stopping treatment, advance directives or euthanasia. These decisions have far-reaching consequences and require close collaboration between the nurse, the patient, the family and the palliative care team.

Educating and raising awareness: The cardiology nurse also has a role to play in raising awareness of the importance of palliative care among other members of the medical team. They can act as a bridge between cardiac care units and palliative care units, facilitating the transfer of knowledge and skills.

Taking care of yourself: Working with a palliative care team can be emotionally challenging. It is essential for nurses to recognise their own emotions, to seek support if necessary, and to practise self-compassion.

The collaboration between the cardiac surgery nurse and palliative care specialists is a powerful alliance, focused on the well-being and dignity of the patient. Each professional brings their own unique skills and perspective, working together with the ultimate aim of providing the best possible quality of life.

Chapter 18:
THE CHALLENGES FACING THE HEALTHCARE SYSTEM AND CARDIAC SURGERY

Understanding the healthcare system and financial challenges

The world of medicine is not only driven by research, innovation and dedication to the cause of human well-being. It is also strongly influenced by the healthcare systems in which it operates, systems often marked by organisational, political and financial complexities. For a healthcare professional, particularly a cardiac surgery nurse, understanding these issues is crucial in order to provide the best possible care while skilfully navigating the maze of bureaucracy and budgetary constraints.

The Global Health System Framework: Each country has its own health system, shaped by decades, even centuries, of policy, tradition and negotiation. Some systems are largely state-funded, others rely on private insurance, and many are a mixture of the two. Knowing the basic structure of your country's healthcare system helps nurses to guide patients and understand the challenges they face.

Financial pressures: The costs of cardiac surgery, as with many advanced medical procedures, are high. This includes everything from surgeons' fees to the cost of medical devices and hospitalisation costs. Patients, their families and sometimes even medical staff can be overwhelmed by these costs, leading to ethical dilemmas about fair access to care.

The role of insurance companies: Insurance companies often play a central role in determining what is covered, at what level, and under what conditions. Nurses often have to work closely with these bodies to ensure optimum cover.

Ethical issues: The question of who receives what treatment, when and how, is deeply rooted in ethical issues. With limited resources, difficult decisions have to be made, sometimes leaving healthcare professionals conflicted between their desire to help and financial realities.

The Importance of Prevention: With the rising cost of healthcare, the importance of prevention has never been more crucial. By educating patients about cardiac risk factors and promoting healthy lifestyles, nurses play a key role in reducing future costs.

Innovation and Cost: While new technologies and surgical methods can offer better results and faster recoveries, they often come with a high price tag. Striking a balance between adopting these innovations and controlling costs is a constant challenge.

Training and Development : Financial challenges also affect continuing education. Institutions can sometimes be reluctant to invest in staff training because of budgetary constraints, potentially jeopardising the quality of care.

Navigating the world of healthcare requires much more than medical skills. It's a delicate balance between delivering quality care, understanding the system, and recognising the ever-present financial challenges. For the cardiac surgery nurse, this means being as comfortable with a scalpel as with a budget.

The influence of health policy on cardiac surgery

The intersection between health policy and cardiac surgery is a fascinating area, marking the convergence between the macroscopic spectrum of government decisions and the micro-reality of operating theatres. The evolution, availability and quality of cardiac surgery in a given region are highly dependent on the priorities, policies and investments defined by political leaders.

Funding and Resource Allocation: Political decisions largely determine the funding allocated to different health sectors. Funds may be allocated for state-of-the-art equipment, specialist cardiology centres or for training specialist staff. The distribution of these resources has a direct impact on the accessibility and quality of cardiac care.

Equal Access to Care: Healthcare policies often define who has access to what types of care. For example, in some systems, advanced cardiac procedures might be reserved for patients with specific insurance or living in certain regions, leaving other patients in precarious situations.

Research and Development : Political initiatives can stimulate or hinder cardiac surgery research. Strong government support for medical research can lead to innovations in surgical techniques, medical devices and medicines.

Standards and regulations: Standards of practice and regulations influence how cardiac surgery is performed. These may include sterility standards, post-operative protocols, or guidelines on the use of certain technologies.

Prevention Programmes: The impact of policy on heart surgery is not only reactive but also preventative. Strong policies on heart disease prevention, such as health education programmes or regulations on junk food advertising, can reduce the need for heart surgery.

International relations: Foreign policies and trade agreements can influence cardiac surgery, particularly in terms of imports of equipment and medicines, or even the exchange of knowledge and training between countries.

Politics and ethics: Sometimes ethical dilemmas arise, such as deciding whether an expensive treatment should be offered universally or reserved for a specific sub-group of patients. These dilemmas are often influenced by political decisions.

Ultimately, health policy shapes the way cardiac surgery is practised, funded and developed. Cardiac surgeons, nurses and other healthcare professionals must not only master their clinical skills, but also understand and, in some cases, influence policy to ensure the best possible care for their patients.

Working with administrators and decision-makers

In the complex world of healthcare, interprofessional collaboration is not limited to interactions between healthcare professionals. It also encompasses the close links between clinical staff, such as nurses and doctors, and administrators or decision-makers, individuals often in charge of logistics, finance, strategy or human resources. This collaboration is essential to ensure optimal patient care while respecting organisational and budgetary constraints.

The Interconnection of Roles: Although the roles of clinicians and administrators are distinct, they are deeply interconnected. Decisions taken by administrators directly influence clinicians' working conditions and the quality of care provided to patients. Conversely, feedback from clinicians is crucial for administrators to make informed decisions.

Open Communication: Transparent communication is the foundation of effective collaboration. Nurses must be able to express their concerns, needs or suggestions, while understanding the budgetary or organisational constraints that administrators have in mind.

Understanding the Issues: To facilitate this collaboration, it is essential that everyone understands each other's issues and challenges. Nurses should have a basic knowledge of management principles, while administrators should be familiar with the clinical context, including the specific challenges of cardiac surgery.

Patient-centred solutions: In any discussion or negotiation, the patient's well-being must remain at the centre of attention. Decisions must always be aimed at improving the quality of care and the patient experience, even if this requires compromises on both sides.

Collaboration forums: Joint committees or working groups including both clinicians and administrators can be set up to discuss specific topics, such as the purchase of new equipment, the improvement of work processes or ongoing training.

Continuing education: Organising workshops or joint training courses can strengthen mutual understanding and improve collaboration. For example, a workshop on the latest innovations in cardiac surgery may be of interest to both specialist nurses and financial managers.

Participation in decision-making: Including nurses in decision-making processes, particularly those that directly affect their clinical practice, strengthens their sense of belonging and motivation. It can also help to identify innovative solutions or anticipate potential problems.

Collaboration between nurses and administrators is not always straightforward, as it involves reconciling sometimes differing visions. However, when this collaboration is successful, it can lead to a significant improvement in patient care, greater professional satisfaction and improved organisational efficiency.

Chapter 19:
CONTINUING EDUCATION AND PROFESSIONAL DEVELOPMENT

The importance of ongoing training

In the medical field and, more specifically, in cardiac surgery, continuing education is not only an imperative, but also a guarantee of the quality of the care provided. It enables professionals, including nurses, to remain at the cutting edge of knowledge, master the latest techniques and guarantee optimum patient care.

Constantly evolving knowledge: Medicine is a constantly evolving science. Research advances, new discoveries are made, and medical recommendations can change. Continuing education helps us to stay informed and up to date, ensuring that patients benefit from the best practices available.

Integration of Technological Innovations: With the emergence of new technologies, such as advanced monitoring devices or innovative surgical techniques, it is essential that nurses become familiar with these tools. Appropriate training ensures that these technologies are used safely and effectively for the benefit of the patient.

Improving clinical skills: Continuing education is not just theoretical. It also includes practical workshops, simulations and on-the-job training to reinforce and perfect nurses' clinical skills.

Strengthening multidisciplinarity: Training courses are often an opportunity for the various players in the medical world to meet and exchange ideas. These interactions enrich each person's practice, promote a better understanding of their respective roles and strengthen collaboration within teams.

Meeting regulatory requirements: In many countries, a certain number of hours of continuing education is required to maintain a licence or professional accreditation. Beyond this obligation, it is also proof of professional commitment.

Professional and personal development: Continuing education also contributes to the professional development of nurses, offering them opportunities for specialisation or career progression. On a personal level, it boosts self-confidence, job satisfaction and a sense of achievement.

Preventing medical errors: Regular training helps to reduce the risk of medical errors by reminding patients of good practice and raising awareness of common errors and pitfalls to be avoided.

Adaptation to Specific Contexts: Cardiac surgery, with its specific features and challenges, requires refined knowledge. Training targeted at this speciality enables us to meet the unique needs of cardiac patients.

In short, continuing education is a cornerstone of the cardiac surgery nursing profession. It embodies the commitment of carers to their patients, their profession and themselves, ensuring optimal quality of care in a constantly evolving field.

Conferences, seminars and relevant workshops

Staying active and informed in the medical field, particularly cardiac surgery, requires regular attendance at conferences, seminars and workshops. These professional gatherings are not only learning opportunities, but also privileged moments to exchange with peers, discuss the latest advances and collaborate on clinical or research issues.

The scope of conferences: There are a multitude of medical conferences, ranging from international cardiology symposia with thousands of participants, to more intimate meetings focusing on specific topics such as new surgical techniques or post-operative management.

Specialised Seminars: Seminars are often more focused and in-depth than a general conference. They may cover specific subjects such as the use of particular technologies, the management of specific complications or the ethical issues involved in heart transplantation.

Practical workshops: Unlike conferences and seminars, which are often theoretical, workshops are practical sessions. They may involve mastering new equipment, surgical simulations or training in patient-nurse communication.

Exchanging and networking: These events are an ideal opportunity to meet colleagues, establish professional contacts and discuss clinical cases or personal experiences. This network can be invaluable for obtaining advice, collaborating on research projects or simply sharing challenges and successes.

Stay Informed: With medicine evolving so rapidly, attending these events is a great way to keep abreast of the latest advances, whether in research, new surgical techniques or clinical recommendations.

Active participation: Many professionals not only attend these events as listeners, but also get actively involved by presenting their research, leading workshops or taking part in round tables. This active participation is an excellent opportunity to make yourself known and to contribute to the professional community.

Training opportunities: For many nurses, these conferences, seminars and workshops can also count as hours of continuing education, required to maintain certain certifications or accreditations.

Challenges and Controversies: These events are also the stage for lively discussions on controversial issues, providing a space for ethical, clinical or even political debate.

International perspective: The major conferences offer an international perspective, enabling us to understand how cardiac surgery is practised in different contexts and cultures.

Taking part in these professional meetings is essential for all cardiac surgery nurses who want to provide the best possible care, while actively contributing to the advancement of their profession.

Mentoring and coaching new nurses

The integration of a new nurse into a department, particularly in a field as demanding and specialised as cardiac surgery, is a delicate moment, both for the professional and for the existing team. Mentoring and coaching are essential tools for ensuring a smooth transition, promoting skills development and strengthening team cohesion.

The Essence of Mentoring : Mentoring is not just technical training. It is a privileged professional relationship in which an experienced nurse, the mentor, guides, supports and advises a newcomer. This relationship is based on trust, exchange and mutual commitment.

Passing on know-how: The field of cardiac surgery is rich in techniques, protocols and specialist knowledge. The mentor guides the new nurse through this complexity, helping them to link theory and practice, hone their skills and adapt to the specificities of the department.

Emotional and Psychological Support: The world of cardiac surgery can be stressful and emotionally demanding. The mentor is there to help the new nurse navigate these sometimes tumultuous waters, offering a listening ear, advice and reassurance.

Integration into the team: The mentor also facilitates the social and professional integration of the new nurse. He or she acts as a mediator, introducing the newcomer to the team, decoding the department's culture and establishing a climate of trust.

Constructive feedback: One of the mentor's essential functions is to provide regular feedback. This feedback, which is both positive and corrective, enables the new nurse to progress, adjust their practices and build up their self-confidence.

Evolution of mentoring: While the mentoring relationship is initially very structured, it evolves over time. As the new nurse gains in autonomy and confidence, the mentor adapts his or her approach, offering more freedom while remaining available for support and advice.

Valuing the role of mentor: Being a mentor is a responsibility, but also a way of recognising know-how and experience. It's an opportunity for experienced nurses to pass on their knowledge, but also to challenge themselves, update their skills and renew their commitment to the profession.

Creating a lasting bond: Mentoring often leads to a lasting professional relationship based on mutual respect and exchange. Mentor and mentee can become colleagues, collaborators or even friends, sharing a common history and a passion for their profession.

Mentoring and coaching new nurses is essential to ensure a successful integration, strengthen team skills and guarantee optimal care for cardiac surgery patients. It's a win-win situation that benefits the mentor, the mentee, the team and, ultimately, the patients.

Chapter 20:
THE BALANCE
WORK-LIFE

Recognising the signs of burnout

In the demanding and fast-paced world of cardiac surgery, it is crucial for nurses and all medical staff to recognise the signs of burnout. Untreated burnout can not only impact the mental and physical health of the individual concerned, but also compromise the quality of care provided to patients.

Physical symptoms: Exhaustion often manifests itself as chronic, insurmountable fatigue, even after a full night's sleep. This fatigue can be accompanied by headaches, muscular pains, sleep disturbances, digestive problems and reduced resistance to infection.

Impaired Cognitive Functions: Decreased concentration, frequent forgetfulness, difficulty in making decisions and prolonged reaction time are all warning signs. In a surgical context, these symptoms can have dramatic consequences.

Emotions and mood: Exhaustion can lead to mood swings, increased irritability, feelings of sadness or depression, feelings of isolation, and reduced personal satisfaction.

Behaviour at work: A lack of interest in work, a drop in motivation, frequent lateness, an increase in medical errors, or a tendency to isolate oneself from colleagues can be signs of burnout.

Changes in Social Relationships: A tendency to isolate, a lack of interest in social activities or hobbies, and a feeling of distance from loved ones can also be revealing.

Negative attitudes: A cynical view of work, a feeling of being overwhelmed, of being trapped in one's job, or doubting the value or meaning of one's work are typical symptoms of burnout.

Risky Behaviours: Some people may develop self-destructive behaviours such as excessive alcohol consumption, drug use, unbalanced eating or other risky behaviours in response to exhaustion.

It is crucial for healthcare professionals, team leaders and even family members to know how to recognise these signs. This enables them to intervene quickly, offer support and, if necessary, direct the person to the appropriate resources. In the medical field, and particularly in cardiac surgery where every gesture counts, taking care of oneself is inseparable from the quality of care provided to patients.

Strategies for maintaining a healthy balance

Healthcare professionals, particularly those working in the demanding environment of cardiac surgery, are often under intense pressure. However, it is essential to maintain a healthy work-life balance to ensure quality care while preserving one's own mental and physical health. Here are some strategies that can help you find and maintain that balance.

1. Prioritisation and Delimitation: It's vital to define your priorities clearly, both professionally and personally. This allows you to devote time to what really matters. Establishing boundaries between work and private life, such as avoiding bringing work home or disconnecting from work emails during holidays, can help preserve this balance.

2. Take time for yourself: It's essential to regularly set aside time for relaxation and leisure. This can be as simple as reading a book, exercising, meditating or spending quality time with loved ones.

3. Stress management: Techniques such as meditation, yoga and deep breathing can be beneficial in reducing stress. It may also be useful to consult a therapist or specialist coach to learn appropriate stress management strategies.

4. Regular exercise: Physical activity is not only good for your physical health, it's also a great way to relieve stress and improve your mood thanks to the release of endorphins.

5. A balanced diet: Proper nutrition supports physical and mental well-being. Eating a balanced diet, drinking enough water and avoiding excess can improve resilience in the face of stress.

6. Sleep: Getting enough quality sleep is essential. Lack of sleep can aggravate stress, reduce cognitive capacity and have a negative impact on health.

7. Establish a Support Network: Having colleagues, friends or family members to talk to and share experiences with can be a great help in decompressing.

8. Ongoing training: Updating skills and learning new methods can reduce professional anxiety and boost self-confidence.

9. Learn to delegate: It's important to recognise that you can't do everything on your own. Delegating certain tasks, whether at work or at home, helps to spread the load more evenly.

10. Take a holiday: It's vital to take breaks, even short ones, to recharge your batteries, rest and come back stronger.

Keeping in mind that there's no shame in asking for help when balance seems elusive is crucial. Whether it's a healthcare professional, a mentor or someone close to you, talking about your feelings and looking for solutions together is often the first step towards a healthy balance.

The importance of support
social and professional

In the tumultuous world of medicine, and particularly in specialities as demanding as cardiac surgery, social and professional support is a lifeline for many professionals. Far from being a simple 'extra', it is a fundamental pillar of well-being, professional effectiveness and longevity in the profession. Let's explore together why this support is so vital.

Social support, whether from family, friends or the community, provides an emotional refuge, a place where nurses can recharge their batteries, express their doubts and frustrations, or share their successes. This type of support has a number of benefits:

- **Resilience in the face of stress**: simply talking to someone you trust about your experiences can reduce the effects of stress. Shared emotions are often easier to manage.
- **Outside perspective**: Friends and family can offer a different point of view, allowing the individual to see things from a new perspective, outside the medical context.
- **Belonging**: Feeling integrated and appreciated within a social group boosts self-esteem and confidence.
- **Balance**: Social interaction outside the workplace helps to maintain a work-life balance, which is essential for mental health.

Professional support, on the other hand, stems from relationships between colleagues, mentors and hierarchical superiors. It's an interconnected network where knowledge, skills and experience are shared.

- **Professional growth**: mentors and experienced colleagues can provide advice, tips and techniques that enrich individual practice.

Challenge Management: Faced with a complex case or an unexpected situation, the team can come together to find solutions, which reduces the feeling of isolation.

Constructive feedback: Honest, benevolent feedback helps you to improve, understand your mistakes and learn from them.

Solidarity: Knowing and being recognised by your peers creates a feeling of belonging to a close-knit group, where helping each other is natural.

Exchanging resources: Whether it's a new training course, a relevant article or an upcoming conference, the professional network is a mine of information.

Support, whether social or professional, is not a luxury: it's a necessity. It brings balance, strength, growth and wellbeing, essential elements for any healthcare professional wishing to provide the best possible care while preserving their own health and passion for their profession.

Chapter 21:
FUTURE PROSPECTS
AND DEVELOPMENT
OF THE PROFESSION

Current and future challenges
cardiac surgery

Cardiac surgery, at the crossroads of medicine, technology and research, is constantly evolving. From its daring beginnings to the technical prowess of today, it has always been at the heart of medical advances. However, despite its successes, this medical speciality faces a series of current and future challenges that it is essential to recognise and address.

Current challenges :
  Increasing patient complexity: As the population ages and co-morbidities increase, patients requiring surgery are often older and have more complex medical conditions.
  Limited resources: In many parts of the world, access to state-of-the-art cardiac surgery facilities remains limited, highlighting inequalities in care.
  Rapid Technological Evolution : Medical technology is advancing at a breakneck pace. While this brings innovations, it also poses challenges in terms of training, adaptation and costs.
  Antimicrobial resistance: The increasing prevalence of drug resistance, particularly in the context of post-operative infections, is a major concern.
Future Challenges :
  Integration of Artificial Intelligence (AI): With the advent of AI, how can these technologies best be integrated to improve diagnosis, intervention and

follow-up, while ensuring that professionals are properly trained?

- **Bioengineering and Transplantation**: Advances in artificial hearts and the cultivation of heart tissue in the laboratory could revolutionise transplantation. However, these advances will require ethical, legal and clinical adjustments.
- **Demographic and epidemiological changes**: The increase in non-communicable diseases, such as obesity, could lead to an increase in heart disease, requiring adequate planning and preparation.
- **Ethics and Patient Autonomy**: As surgical options become more varied and complex, how can we ensure informed, patient-centred decision-making?
- **Impact of Climate Change**: Extreme weather events, pollution and other environmental factors can influence heart health. How can cardiac surgery adapt to these new challenges?

The ability to anticipate and navigate these challenges will define the future of cardiac surgery. This will require interdisciplinary collaboration, continuing education and a commitment to innovation to ensure that the specialty continues to offer cutting-edge care while evolving with the times.

Advanced career opportunities for nurses (nurse practitioner, clinical specialist, etc.)

Nursing is one of the pillars of modern medicine. While the fundamental role of the nurse is to provide direct patient care, the nursing field has diversified and specialised considerably over time, offering many advanced career opportunities. Thanks to these specialisations, nurses can not only broaden their clinical scope, but also influence health policy, research, education and management.

1. Nurse Practitioner (NP):

The nurse practitioner is a highly qualified healthcare professional, capable of making diagnoses, prescribing treatments, and independently managing certain pathologies. There are several specialities for NPs, including :

- Family care NP
- IP in acute care
- IP in paediatrics
- IP in geriatrics
- IP in psychiatry/mental health

2. Clinical Nurse Specialist (CNS):

The ICS is an expert in a specific clinical specialty. They play a central role in training new nurses, implementing care protocols and improving the quality of care.

3. Nurse Anaesthetist :

Trained specifically to administer anaesthesia, this nurse works closely with anaesthetists, surgeons and other healthcare professionals to ensure patient safety during surgical procedures.

4. Nurse researcher :

Some nurses decide to go into clinical or basic research. They may work on epidemiological studies, clinical trials or laboratory research, thereby contributing to the advancement of health knowledge.

5. Public Health Nurse :

Focused on communities, public health nurses work on disease prevention, health promotion and health education for the population.

6. Nurse Legal Consultant:

Bridging the gap between law and medicine, this nurse offers expertise in legal matters related to medical practice, whether in litigation, malpractice or consultation for laws and regulations.

7. Nurse Educator:
Whether in universities or nursing schools, the nurse educator plays a key role in training future generations of nurses.

8. Nurse in Management and Leadership:
With additional training in management, nurses can take on leadership roles within healthcare facilities, managing teams, budgets and projects.

9. Computer Nurse :
At the intersection of health and technology, this nurse specializes in health-related information systems, helping to set up and optimize electronic medical records and other technologies.

These advanced careers often require additional training, specific certifications and in-depth clinical experience. But they offer nurses the opportunity to have an even greater impact on patient health and the healthcare system as a whole.

The role of the nurse in prevention and cardiac education

Nurses play a vital role in the care of heart patients. In addition to direct care, their mission also encompasses prevention and patient education. This approach aims to equip patients with the knowledge and skills they need to manage their heart health, reduce the associated risks and improve their quality of life.

1. Healthy lifestyle education:
The nurse raises patients' awareness of modifiable cardiac risk factors, such as smoking, a sedentary lifestyle and an unbalanced diet. They offer practical advice on how to adopt a healthier lifestyle, encouraging regular physical activity, a balanced diet and smoking cessation.

2. Symptoms awareness :

The nurse teaches patients to recognise the warning signs of a heart problem, such as chest pain, shortness of breath or palpitations. This can lead to early treatment and avoid complications.

3. Medication management:

The nurse explains the role, benefits and potential side effects of each drug prescribed. He or she stresses the importance of compliance in order to maximise the benefits of treatment and prevent complications.

4. Post-operative follow-up :

After cardiac surgery, the nurse educates the patient on wound care, gradual resumption of activities, monitoring for signs of infection or complications, and any adjustments to treatment.

5. Support Groups:

Some nurses may facilitate or refer patients to support groups where they can share experiences, support each other and learn new strategies for managing their illness.

6. Secondary prevention :

For patients who have already suffered a cardiac event, the nurse stresses the importance of secondary prevention, i.e. preventing recurrences. This involves regular medical monitoring, taking prescribed medication and adopting a heart-healthy lifestyle.

7. Liaison with other health professionals:

Nurses work in collaboration with other professionals, such as cardiologists, nutritionists, physiotherapists or psychologists, in order to offer holistic care tailored to each patient.

Nurses play a central role in cardiac prevention and education. As they are often the patient's first point of contact, nurses have the ability to positively influence behaviour, encourage patient autonomy in the management of their disease, and make a significant contribution to the prevention of cardiovascular disease.

Chapter 22:
CONCLUSION

THE NOBILITY
OF THE NURSING PROFESSION
IN CARDIAC SURGERY

Being a cardiac surgery nurse means choosing to stand on the borderline between the fragility of human life and the genius of modern medicine. It means embracing a vocation that combines science, technology, compassion and dedication. This profession, charged with emotion and responsibility, is the epitome of nobility in the medical world.

1. Save the Heart, Symbol of Life :
The heart, the central pump that gives life to every part of our body, is a sacred organ in many cultures. Protecting and caring for the heart is to touch the very essence of life. Cardiac surgery nurses play an active part in this mission, with unrivalled devotion and skill.

2. Knowledge that combines technical expertise and humanity:
Nurses specialising in this field have extensive technical know-how. But their technical skills cannot mask the humanity that lies at the heart of their practice. Each patient is unique, and nurses deploy boundless empathy to understand, reassure and support them.

3. Courage under pressure :
Emergencies are frequent in cardiac surgery. In these critical moments, nurses show remarkable resilience, maintaining their calm, lucidity and precision to ensure the best possible chances of success.

4. Ongoing commitment to patient well-being :
Beyond the operating theatre, nurses play a crucial role in

the patient's recovery and rehabilitation. Their commitment does not end with surgery, but continues with monitoring, education and emotional support, reflecting an unwavering determination to see every patient return to a full and healthy life.

5. Respectful collaboration :
The nobility of the profession is also expressed in the nurse's ability to work in harmony with a multidisciplinary team. Mutual respect, listening and sharing knowledge are essential to providing optimal care.

6. An Unshakeable Ethic :
Faced with ethical dilemmas and the challenges of modern medicine, the cardiac surgery nurse remains a guardian of the fundamental principles of the profession: benevolence, justice, autonomy and non-harmfulness.

7. Constant evolution :
Cardiac surgery is a constantly evolving field. Nurses show a thirst for learning, adapting to new technologies and innovative methods, while preserving the human aspect of care.

Cardiac surgery nursing is not just a profession; it is a vocation, a call to serve, to surpass oneself, to touch lives in a profound way. The nobility of this profession lies not only in its technical skills, but above all in its immeasurable passion, devotion and love for humanity.

Continuing to evolve
to serve patients better

The medical world, like a living organism, is constantly changing. Today's medicine, with its technological advances and discoveries, is radically different from that of a few decades ago. Faced with this unbridled dynamic, healthcare professionals, and cardiac surgery nurses in particular, have a heavy responsibility: to continue to evolve in order to better serve their patients.

Development through continuing education :
Learning never really stops for nurses. New surgical techniques, innovative medicines, cutting-edge equipment... All require regular training to ensure safe and effective interventions. This never-ending quest for knowledge is fuelled by a deep desire to provide the best possible care.

Adaptability to Technology:
The digital age has profoundly changed the healthcare landscape. Electronic patient records, telemedicine, remote monitoring devices are just a few examples of how technology has intruded into daily practice. The modern nurse embraces these tools, not as substitutes, but as complements that improve the quality and precision of care.

Active Listening and Communication :
As the world becomes increasingly noisy, the art of listening becomes a precious treasure. By listening to their patients, nurses can pick up on nuances and details that might escape a standard medical examination. This active listening, coupled with effective communication, builds a relationship of trust between patient and carer.

Humanising care:
With the influx of technological innovations, it is crucial not to lose sight of the human aspect of care. Every patient is unique, with his or her own story, hopes and fears. By recognising and honouring this individuality, nurses add a dimension of empathy and compassion, essential for holistic healing.

Interprofessional collaboration:
The medical world is interconnected. Cardiac surgery nurses work closely with surgeons, cardiologists, anaesthetists and other professionals. This collaboration,

based on mutual respect, ensures that the patient benefits from comprehensive care.

Ethical reflection:

Faced with complex medical dilemmas, nurses are often called upon to reflect ethically, placing the patient's well-being at the heart of every decision.

Continuing to evolve to better serve patients is not just a professional necessity, it's a moral commitment. It's a promise that every nurse makes, not only to their patients but also to themselves: to never stop learning, listening and innovating for the well-being of all.

Encouragement and advice for future nurses in the field

The path you have decided to embark on is one of the noblest and most rewarding there is. Cardiac surgery is a cutting-edge field that demands not only exceptional technical skills but also a profound sense of humanity. As nurses, you will be the guarantors of the quality of care provided to patients, from the moment they cross the hospital's threshold until they make a full recovery. Here are a few words of encouragement and advice to help you on your way.

1. Believe in your mission:

You will play an essential role in every patient's journey to recovery. Your contribution, although sometimes underestimated, is fundamental. Always remember that your work has a profound impact on the lives of the people you care for.

2. Never stop learning:

Medicine evolves rapidly, as does technology. Invest in continuing education to stay at the forefront of your field and ensure the best possible care for your patients.

3. Cultivate Empathy:
Technical skills are essential, but so is the ability to understand and connect emotionally with patients. Your compassion and empathy will often be patients' lifeline in difficult times.

4. Work together:
Cardiac surgery is a team effort. Learn to work closely with surgeons, anaesthetists, dieticians and other healthcare professionals. Together, you can provide comprehensive and holistic care.

5. Take care of yourself:
Working in cardiac surgery can be stressful and exhausting. To take care of others, you must first take care of yourself. Find ways to decompress, whether through hobbies, exercise or meditation.

6. Seek Support:
Whether it's mentors, colleagues or professional support groups, surround yourself with people who can offer advice, reassurance and different perspectives.

7. Don't be afraid of failure:
You will make mistakes, just like everyone else. The important thing is to learn from these mistakes and use them as an opportunity for growth.

8. Keep the Passion:
What drew you to this field in the first place was a passion for helping others. Never forget that spark, as it will guide you through even the most difficult times.

9. Be Proud:
No matter what obstacles you encounter, know that you are doing incredibly important work. Every day you have the opportunity to change lives, and that's something to be proud of.

Cardiac surgery nursing is a unique blend of science, art and humanity. By cultivating both your technical skills and your ability to connect with patients, you will make an invaluable difference. Good luck and welcome to this wonderful adventure!

Glossary of medical terms

A glossary of medical terms is vast and can include thousands of entries. Here is a non-exhaustive list of some commonly used medical terms, with brief definitions:

- **Anemia**: decrease in the number of red blood cells or the quantity of haemoglobin in the blood.
- **Biopsy**: removal of a tissue sample for microscopic examination.
- **Cyanosis**: Bluish discolouration of the skin due to a lack of oxygen in the blood.
- **Dyspnoea**: Difficulty breathing or shortness of breath.
- **Electrocardiogram (ECG):** Recording of the heart's electrical activity.
- **Fibrosis**: Excessive formation of fibrous tissue, often following inflammation or injury.
- **Glycaemia**: concentration of glucose in the blood.
- **Hypertension:** High blood pressure.
- **Immunology**: Study of the immune system and its responses to various pathogens.
- **Jaundice**: yellowing of the skin and eyes due to an increase in bilirubin in the blood.
- **Keratin:** A protein found in the skin, nails and hair.
- **Leukocytes** : White blood cells involved in defending the body against infection.
- **Metabolism**: All the chemical reactions that take place in the body to maintain life.
- **Neoplasia**: abnormal growth of cells, which can lead to a tumour.
- **Oncology**: Study and treatment of tumours.
- **Pathogen**: Organism or agent capable of causing disease.
- **Quadrant** : Division of an anatomical area into four parts, often used to describe the location of abdominal pain.

- **Remission**: Reduction or disappearance of the signs and symptoms of an illness.
- **Serum**: The liquid part of the blood which remains after coagulation.
- **Tachycardia**: Accelerated heart rate.
- **Ulcer:** open lesion, usually painful, which forms on the skin or mucous membranes.
- **Vascularisation**: Supply of blood to a tissue or organ.
- **WBC:** White Blood Cells.
- **Xenograft**: transplant of tissues or organs from a different species.
- **Yoga: A** practice that combines postures, breathing exercises and meditation to promote physical and mental health.
- **Shingles**: Viral disease characterised by painful skin eruptions along a nerve.

This is a limited selection of medical terms, and the medical field is so vast that it would be impossible to cover them all here. If you are looking for specific terms or more information on a particular subject, please let us know!